Goodbye Back Pain

A SUFFERERS' GUIDE TO FULL BACK RECOVERY

DR. LEONARD FAYE

UPDATED 2ND EDITION

ISBN: 1-4196-9144-9
ISBN-13: 9781419691447

Visit www.booksurge.com to order additional copies.

ACKNOWLEDGEMENTS

In the first edition of this book which was written in 1990, I acknowledged the helpers I needed to fulfill a goal of informing back pain sufferers, so that they could become informed, health care consumers. If it wasn't for Ron Baron and Dick Weaver of Tale Weaver Publishing, I would have been unpublished and very frustrated. We have reused my son, Michael Fayes' photographs of Neal Hitchens and Charity Staley in this edition.

I wish to thank those chiropractic colleagues who have joined the paradigm shift away from trying to realign the spine, and over to achieving restoration of locomotor function of the spine and extremities. These doctors realize they are part of a team of professionals, dedicated to helping back pain sufferers, get well. The American Back Society is the platform and melting pot, in the USA, that allows inter professional exchange of research, and therefore prevents ignorance and bias, that used to prevent patients from getting the most effective and harmless treatments.

I thank Dr. Mark King and Dr. Corey Campbell of MPI, for reviewing this work and continuing the evolution of teaching seminars to Chiropractors and chiropractic students all over the world.

I also wish to thank all the patients who presented the problems that stimulated me to continue improving our methods and broadening our approach to lower back pain, which has so many causes, all requiring specific diagnosis and treatment.

TABLE OF CONTENTS

To Bernadette,

my loving wife

and best friend.

INTRODUCTION

"Life is Movement................Movement is Life"

Your back hurts!

You can't work and you can't relax and enjoy yourself.

It is difficult to sit; it's even worse getting up. Bend? Walk? Run? Make love? Pure torture.

As an episodal, back pain, sufferer you are not alone. Each year in the United States, millions of people suffer from a multitude of conditions associated with back ailments. Back pain is as common as the common cold, but with this big difference:

YOU CAN STOP BACK PAIN!

It is estimated that back pain-related problems are costing the American public $65 billion annually. Even at that enormous cost, it would be money well spent if a cure could be guaranteed. Unfortunately, very few people find any kind of long-lasting relief.

By the time the "classic, back pain, sufferer" is around 35 years old, he or she has already been to many practitioners with few lasting results. For this person, there was usually a history of a late teen or early twenties incident which caused severe back pain.

If the sufferer sought a doctor's advice, the recommendation was usually to treat the pain with pain killers, rest and respect until it went away. Every year or so, the pain would flare up after some new incident, but each time the discomfort seemed to get worse from doing less. Different doctors would be consulted and all the arthritic diseases would be ruled out.

Because the disease had not progressed to a point of requiring surgical intervention, the orthopedist would prescribe physiotherapy and plant the concept to return when surgery was necessary for ultimate relief. His attitude towards physiotherapy would be lukewarm at best and far from encouraging. Rarely would manipulation be recommended even though U.S Govt. publications reported this therapy was the therapy of choice at this stage.

Inevitably, this poor sufferer had friends who knew of a chiropractor, osteopath, acupuncturist, masseur, hypnotist, or herbalist who could cure back pain in one easy visit. The sufferer probably went to anyone who might be able to help, as it was obvious the medical approach was yielding few results. There are more than 85 million back pain sufferers in the United States alone who can attest to that fact!

Because this developing condition is episodic it naturally has its good and bad periods. Almost any treatment during a pain episode will succeed to some extent. However, most treatments will not prevent further episodes. In some cases the sufferer gets well in spite of the treatments they receive.

Back pain is a symptom. The disease is a process of disc and joint erosion combined with irregular outgrowths of bone spurs and calcified ligaments combined with deconditioned or hyper active muscles that develop abnormal contraction patterns. The spinal cord and its branches eventually get involved and become diseased. Back pain sufferers can experience occasional pain from age 18 to 40 and be unaware of the process in progress.

THE KEY TO LONG TERM RESULTS IS FOUND IN THE TREATMENT GIVEN AFTER THE PAIN IS CLEARED. The

Chapter One

The Causes of Back Pain

For every action there is a reaction; and for every cause there is an effect.

Communicate Your Symptoms

If you currently have back pain, it is vitally important for you to understand the causes clearly, or be able to describe in detail the various symptoms to your doctor. Back pain can be associated with kidney, gall bladder, pancreas, metastatic cancer, abdominal aortic disease as well as spinal disorders. Vague descriptions will lead to a poor understanding by your doctor and will only delay the correct treatment. If you can articulate all of your symptoms, you can help your doctor help you to get better faster.

Most doctors would agree that a thorough consultation and a carefully recorded case history can almost always guide them to the correct diagnosis. However some doctors, because of their specialty and training, limit themselves to their particular concept as to the causes of back pain. No matter what you tell them, they are going to prescribe the same treatments they always do. For example, an acupuncturist is going to stick needles in the meridians that they think, when blocked, cause back pain or a herbalist will give you herbs known to relieve back pain. There are so many known causes of back pain that getting a biased view often delays treating the correct condition.

There are unique causes to all bad backs and no single treatment system succeeds for everyone. The less the doctor or therapist asks you, the more likely you will be slotted into a system. Beware of the doctor that does not listen and asks specific questions about your back pain: you may become a guinea pig in a treatment mill. Make sure you are treated, as the individual you are.

It is amazing that most people lose their memories when they enter the examination room in a doctors' office. They also become monosyllabic and drop all the descriptive words that could better help the doctor comprehend their condition.

Don't take along a written list (the doctor may peg you as a "neurotic"), but make sure you have a list of your symptoms in your mind. Usually the physical examination and x-rays are only necessary to confirm the diagnosis and to rule out a few rare possibilities.

I can recall treating a non-English speaking patient without an interpreter. He had described where he "used to" get leg pain in minute detail, and I mistakenly thought he was presently suffering from this pain. It turned out after a few weeks he had been describing a pain in his leg he used to get all the time, but never experienced after he strained his back. I had missed the "used to" in my translation of his French. Fortunately, once we began communicating on the same level, I was able to solve his problem.

Even if there is no language barrier, don't tell the doctor you have "a hitch in your get along" or "a pain in your back". Describe exactly where they are. Describe the difference between a sharp or dull pain, a constant or intermittent one. Make certain your doctor knows precisely what you are feeling even if he is too busy to investigate thoroughly. Keep in mind that doctors are human too. It might be difficult for your family doctor to become interested in your back problem when a previous patient was seriously depressed, or had to be told that he or she had a terminal illness.

Remember, a major part of your ability to alleviate back pain is your ability to communicate with your doctor.

How Your Spine Works

To identify the cause of your back problem, it is essential to first understand how the human back works. Once you have a clear picture, you'll be better able to recognize the four major causes of back pain. In a later chapter, you will be able to determine what is causing your back pain and then be able to seek the right advice and treatment.

The spine has three major functions:

1. To support the torso
2. To protect the spinal cord
3. To enable the body to move smoothly in multiple directions

Humans are the only creatures on earth who consistently walk upright upon two legs. Because we are working against gravitational force, there is more stress on our spinal joints, especially in the lower lumbar area. For this reason, we as a species are more prone to back–related problems.

It is important to understand the functional mechanics of the back. As an example, imagine that your backbone functions as a bicycle chain. When it's running properly, you can go up hills, across town, or just run along carefree mile after mile. But if you are trying to get around on a chain with several links which are locked or frozen together, you are in a world of hurt.

As with a bicycle chain, if the chain of 24 individual bones and over 75 joints which link your spine together are in any way impaired (not able to move properly), there will be abnormal wear and tear on your back and body. To complicate the issue, our brain can achieve the movement it desires to occur by recruiting other joints that are not designed for the job and produce repetitive strains on the compensated joints. For example, you could bend over to touch your toes by overstretching the low back, because your hip joints are not able to flex fully or your hamstring muscles are too short.

The inability to flex your ankle fully will affect how you will move your back.

These adaptations to faulty mechanics in one joint causing a compensatory movement in another area is the way a closed circuit of multiple joints all dependant on each other works. Otherwise if we leaned our head to one side and other joints below didn't react immediately we would fall over. For every movement we make the prime movers contract and the resisting muscles relax. These movement patterns have been studied and your practitioner should be able to see if you have normal or abnormal movement patterns.

The spine and all the joints involved with locomotion must be able to move. This movement must be in the correct order of motion, recruitment patterns, in order to prevent episodal back pain and the slow degeneration of the joints, called Osteoarthritis. Treating just the pain (inflammation), is the main reason surgeons can wait patiently for spines to degenerate, to the point they need surgical intervention. Function needs to be restored as well.

How Your Spine Is Put Together

The spine is composed of three basic parts:

1. The bony framework consisting of vertebrae and joints
2. The spinal cord and exiting nerves
3. The soft tissues: muscles, ligaments, discs, fascia, blood vessels

The spinal column has five transitional zones from the head to the tailbone. Two columns run the full length; and although these columns are joined together, they have separate functions. The front part which faces the inside of your body is responsible for support. It consists of block-like structures that are named the Body of the Vertebra.

Single discs lie between each body. Each disc is jelly-like in the center and is surrounded by a wall of strong fibers that keep it together. The wall of webbed fibers are attached around, above and below to the bodies. Thus, the disc is secured between the two bodies.

The vertebral arch makes up the back part of your vertebra. It is so named because it forms an arch that houses the spinal cord. Attached to the vertebral arch are the upper and lower joints that allow movement in your back.

To complete this picture of the basic spinal structure, refer to Diagram 1 showing a pair of vertebrae (The Basic Motion Unit) on page 10.

In order to understand how your spine is designed, it may be simpler to just imagine a stack of blocks. Think of the front column made up of blocks with discs in between, and two columns on both sides to the rear composed of slippery joints. We call each of these sets of two blocks a motion unit. The joint surfaces are called facets.

Mother Nature has given us ligaments to keep these little stacks from falling apart while moving. Ligaments work much like tiny ropes to guide the movement, while muscles contract to cause the movement.

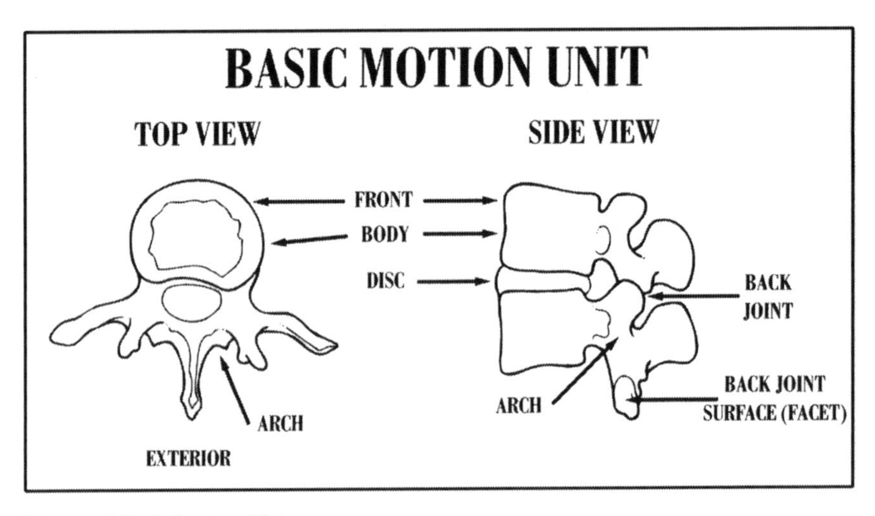

Diagram 1 Basic Motion Unit

Finally, our spinal column curves in a lazy "S" shape from front to back. This curve is not only normal it allows for optimal function. If the spine curves from side to side the spinal column adapts to a coil to increase its' ability to tolerate a heavy load. Of course too much curve or too little curve will impair movement. If x-rays are not taken perfectly, any misplacement will project on to the film as a curve. This becomes a distortion of projection and doesn't really exist in the person being x-rayed. Unfortunately this is not an uncommon error if the radiology technician is not paying very particular attention.

Four Basic Causes of Episodal Back Pain

With a basic grasp of how the spine is set up, you will be better able to understand the four basic causes of back pain, which are:

1. MECHANICAL
This category is divided into two groups: **dysfunctional**, resulting from a repetitive job like a brick-layers or check-out person; and **traumatic**, resulting from an injurious incident such as a car accident or a fall.

2. DEGENERATIVE
This refers to pain caused by unhealthy, weak and broken-down tissue which is not able to provide the necessary support and movement.

3. SYSTEMIC
This category includes Rheumatoid and Gouty Arthritis, Osteoporosis, Anemia, Allergies, Metastatic Cancer, and a few very rare conditions.

4. STRESS-INDUCED
Dr. Hans Selye M.D., Ph.D. wrote a lay book called "The Stress of Life". In his many years of research at McGill University in Montreal, Canada; he fathered the discovery of the physiology of "Stress". One effect of stress is chronic muscle contractions that cause a restriction of the spinal joints and instigate a non-stop pain cycle.

Let's now discuss these four groups in more detail, with the purpose of seeing where you fit. Sometimes, patients are dealing with more than one of these classifications.

MECHANICAL BACK PAIN

Chances are that your disorder falls into this category. 90% of people suffering from back ailments have a mechanical cause that creates inflammation, muscle spasm and pain. The main mechanical disorders that lead to back pain are the irregular motion of joints, irregular muscle patterns, foot, ankle and leg dysfunctions, shortened muscles and muscle deconditioning, and of course physical injury.

MECHANICAL DYSFUNCTION

You have already learned that the basic unit of your back is a motion unit. Most motion units consist of two vertebra connected by a disc and the two posterior superior and posterior inferior joints.

The disc acts like a rubber, ball bearing, allowing the vertebra to move because the ball can bend and twist along with the vertebral joints. From a mechanical point of view, it is extremely important for the disc to twist and bend without restriction, and for the two joints to be able to slide in the directions necessary for smooth locomotion of your body. If there is any breakdown in the joints' ability to flex forward, extend backward, rotate to the left and right, or bend sideways to the left and right, then you have the first stage of mechanical dysfunction. In other words, you will experience pain if a joints' ability to move is in any way impaired. Motion in the lower back is dependent upon flexibility of the pelvis joints. These joints allow the pelvis to transfer mechanical forces from the upper body to the low back down through the pelvis, hip joints to the legs and into the feet, to the ground. If the pelvic joints, called the sacroiliac joints, are not able to accommodate flexion and extension, then you will feel stress and pain when attempting these movements. The entire spine and pelvis must also be mobile on the hip joints, much like the universal joint to the axle of a car, so that the car can move forward or backward. Chapter Two will offer simple tests so you can determine if you have normal hip function or not.

The following is an example of impaired hip functioning. Some years ago, an article appeared in a popular magazine written by a chronic back pain sufferer who had been almost everywhere in an attempt to find relief. The gist of his story was that after many years of suffering with debilitating back pain and a limp, he was finally cured when an Osteopath pulled his leg and he felt a suction-like "pop" in his hip joint. The back pain cleared because the faulty hip joint mechanics traumatizing his lower back had been corrected. Many patients have experienced such relief after a hip manipulation or a foot and ankle manipulation.

If your ankle joints are weakened in any way (if they collapse inward rather than stay upright as they should), then the forces of rotation which occur in the leg transfer up to the knees, hip and sacroiliac joints, produce a very damaging force in the lumbar spine. The result is inflammation and pain around the posterior joints.

These pronated or supinated ankle joints may or may not cause foot pain. Usually these ankle dysfunctions are corrected by good orthotic inserts into the shoes. Orthotics will be discussed in a later chapter on treatment.

Muscles not maintained properly through regular use lose their flexibility and function, and are vulnerable to sudden injury. A recent MRI study done in Australia demonstrated that chronic low back pain sufferers have muscle wasting and fatty degeneration of the very important core muscles called the Multifidus muscles. If you sit a lot, muscles become shortened due to disuse, misuse or the lack of proper stretching and strengthening exercises.

How many times have you heard the story about someone who simply bent over to pick up a piece of paper only to injure their back? I hear this story constantly in my practice. It has probably happened to you. I even had one patient who was bending over to sit on the toilet when the pain and spasm struck! These all-to-frequent occurrences happen because we sit too much. Too much sitting causes the large muscles behind the thighs and the small interior muscles in the lower back to shorten and weaken. When these muscles are suddenly asked to lengthen by the postural change during bending and stooping, they tend to emit a very sharp pain and go into spasms. Stretching and strengthening exercises are vital to avoid this common cause of back pain.

It is significant to note that poor posture is one of the major causes of mechanical back disorders. Postural stress is frequently the result of sitting for a long time in a poor position, or standing or bending incorrectly while working. Several years ago, Lyman Johnston, a Canadian chiropractor, invented the Posture-O-Meter. This device could determine whether a person was standing with the force of gravity being correctly carried by the spinal column. If the persons' weight was too far behind the proper center of gravity, the Posture-O-Meter assigned a number to rate the so-called "Posterior Gravity Line". When a group of people were screened it was shown that over 90% of the back pain sufferers carried their weight to far behind the established normal gravity line. One of our tests in this book actually catches this problem without the use of the Posture-O-Meter.

Sitting improperly is the worst thing you can do to your back, and one of the easiest postures to correct. If you slump in your seat, day after day, the normal hollow that should exist between your back and the chair disappears. The shoulders tend to follow suit and slump forward as well.

What occurs is a reverse of natures' natural curve in the lower back. Instead of there being a space between your lower back and the chair, the hollow disappears and your back touches the chair. In fact a space appears between your shoulders and the chair. Constant posture reversing puts an incredible stretch on the ligaments and allows the lower back discs to creep backwards and bulge. This creeping action happens in about twenty minutes and accounts for the back sufferer who suddenly can't rise from an airplane, sofa or theater seat. Thus, you can not only get a stretched, painful ligament, you can also get a bulging disc which is also very painful.

When people with this type of posture rise from a sitting position, they compensate by throwing their heads forward, which further increases the reversal of the natural curve. Finally the day comes when they try to rise and straighten up and they are unable to do so.

Mechanical dysfunction, trauma, and the chronic stress of poor posture can be the forerunner of the degenerative disease process. Recognize you have an opportunity to prevent and slow down the aging process. Joints that move and are not overused don't degenerate. Research has shown that locked joints and joints that move off their proper axis of movement ---Degenerate.

INJURY --- STRAIN AND SPRAIN

The irregular motion of joints, leg problems, imbalanced muscles and fascia adhesions are the main mechanical disorders that lead to back pain. Added to these are the physical forces of injury that result in sprain/ strain pain immediately. These types of traumatic problems can be described in many cases as adding injury to mechanical insult.

One thing the medical community agrees on, when it comes to back pain, is that strains and sprains are the most common cause of pain over anything else. Lay persons often confuse these two types of injury. However, there is a big difference between the two.

Strain, the lesser of the two, results when muscles and tendons are stretched beyond their normal capacity. The shooting, severe pain produces more muscle spasm. The spasm also restricts blood circulation, so that the natural toxic by-products of normal muscle activity are not carried away in the bloodstream. This pain cycle can last for days or weeks. In some cases a "Trigger Point" develops and symptoms are experienced in a distant tissue. Trigger Points are most commonly found in muscles that are inhibited from taking part in a sequence of movements.

These areas of referred pain, numbness and weakness have been fully mapped and displayed on charts, for all to be aware of.

A Trigger Point will assure that the back pain persists and usually causes the development of pain further away from the strained muscle. This new pain can be intensified when the trigger point is stretched or pressed upon. These trigger points can also send numbness and tingling to the distant point in the leg or buttock. Trigger Points are a common complication of strained lower back muscles.

Back sprain is different from strain in that it occurs when there is a tearing of the ligaments, tendons or muscle fibers. Lower back muscles do not strain as often as ligaments sprain. During forward bending E.M.G. studies show us the back muscles become relaxed and gravity makes you fall into a bent position. At this point you are hanging on your ligaments which are very vulnerable to sprain, especially if you are twisted to one side and try to lift at the same time.

For this reason, you should bend your knees before you bend over to lift. With bent knees your back remains more upright and allows the back muscles to remain contracted, preventing the low back ligaments from spraining. If you don't pivot fully on your hip joints, you hang on your ligaments sooner than normal. And if the weight of your upper body plus the weight you are lifting is too much, a sprain will inevitably occur to the lower back joint ligaments. Sprains hurt immediately and get worse as the local swelling occurs over the next 24 hours, Hence the next day you are in more pain. Fluid and the chemicals released from the injured tissues collects, producing pressure and irritation on the nerves, and so another source of pain develops. Then Nature steps in: the muscles around the area contract and hold to form a natural splint around the joint sprain and spasms occur over a wider range as more muscle bundles contract. The bigger the sprain the greater the muscle splinting; the injured joint is prevented from moving.

Sprains can occur from the repetitive strain of poor posture, occupational positions and actions, injury from accidents, unexpected movements such as missing a step, or even sneezing.

Sprains are far more serious than strains and normally take much more time to heal.

Occasionally the Piriformis muscle in the buttock area is strained. This short but very strong muscle is a hip rotator and a poor stabilizer of the pelvis when we stand on one leg. If the brain asks the piriformis to do the stabilizing job of the gluteus maximus muscle, then we know there is poor communication from the brain and mechanical dysfunction is occurring. The piriformis muscle is located right where you sit on your buttock. When it is in spasm it can trap the Sciatic nerve and cause severe leg pain that mimics Sciatic Neuritis. If you have strained your Piriformis muscle, sitting is painful and you probably keep pushing your thumb into your buttock muscles to ease the spasm. You may feel there is something wrong with your hip. Bowling is often the activity that strains the Piriformis or walking up a lot of stairs can also do it.

One last note on mechanical disorders: if the condition is allowed to persist, your brain will learn to interpret the accompanying restrictions as your normal. You can become stuck in the compensation indefinitely. Reversing these conditioned patterns requires specific, rehabilitation, balance exercises few doctors prescribe. However it should be noted that Chiropractors and Physiotherapists are rehabilitating patients with these methods, routinely now. We will discuss these methods in much more detail in a later chapter.

Degenerative Back Pain

Although this is a separate cause of back pain, in most cases degenerative back pain is actually a progression of the mechanical disorders. It has to do with wear and tear. If something is working incorrectly, then it usually wears out more quickly than if it had been working correctly. A simple comparison is the front end of your car. If the wheels are misaligned, then the tires will wear out more quickly, as well as unevenly.

Dr. David Cassidy, one of the first Chiropractors to do research, removed the front legs from mice and forced them to be bipedal by placing their food and water up high, on the side of the cages. In a matter of a few months, the new strain on the sacroiliac joints caused advanced degenerative changes. Their sacroiliac joints were not designed for bipedal locomotion.

Wear, tear and exercise can frequently be bedfellows. I will never forget the largest, calcium, bone spurs I ever saw on an x-ray that were jutting out from a pair of lumbar vertebrae. The patient was an army, physical education instructor who led an aerobics class four times a day almost every day of the week. His back pain only came on when he had a few days off duty. This pattern lasted for years. When he worked at exercising and stretching he got relief from the pain. During vacations he suffered with a bad back.

The explanation of his problem involves a paradox. It has been shown that exercising with faulty mechanics establishes a corresponding, compensating, muscle splint. This natural splint needs a daily workout to be stimulated into its' supporting role. In the meantime, because the mechanics are faulty, the production of a more permanent splint in the form of calcium spurs is stimulated. The wear and tear and low grade inflammation, eventually lead to the build up of calcium deposits, which are the little spurs that jut out from the edges of the joints and bodies of the vertebrae. These can become quite large at more than a quarter of an inch or six millimeters.

The moral of the story is to make sure you are exercising with normal, mechanical movement. All the joints in your spinal column and the rest of your locomotor system must be mobile with no lock ups. In the chiropractic world these lock ups are called "Subluxations" and other professions call them "Blockages" or "Dysfunction".

Exercise can be a double-edged sword, and using exercise for pain relief can lead to degenerative changes sooner than you think. The joints which aren't functioning properly will be compensated for without you realizing the process is progressing. Someone has to examine you to determine the areas of joint loss of movement and their compensatory muscle patterns.

With this advice, this cause of degeneration can be corrected. Luckily this type of degeneration is accompanied by painful inflammation. Pain can be regarded as an early, warning system.

It is like hitting your thumb with a hammer. It becomes painful to touch after the trauma, whereas normally you could squeeze your thumb without pain. Compressing or stretching inflamed areas hurts. The inflamed areas of your back can't take the pressure of compression or stretching either. That is why it hurts to bend forward, backwards or to the side.

The whole degenerative process is full of such painful scenarios, and in most cases, much unnecessary suffering.

Systemic Back Pain

This category refers to diseases that affect the whole body, including the joints of the spinal column.

Arthritic Conditions

Foremost on the list of systemic disorders is Rheumatoid Arthritis.

Let's look at these terms separately. Rheumatic diseases affect the connective tissues of the body, often striking the spine as well as the extremity joints. Arthritis (from arthra = joint and itis = inflammation) literally means the inflammation of a joint.

Inside the affected joints, the cartilage thins out and the joint space narrows with the deterioration, as the disease progresses. This degeneration causes the release of chemicals which prolong and advance the condition.

Rheumatoid Arthritis is considered an autoimmune disease. That is, the systems anti-bodies, which normally protect against disease, go berserk and gradually begin eating away at the soft tissues of the joints. Stress, nutrition and emotional factors play a large part in generating this condition.

Blood tests can monitor the rheumatoid activity and rheumatologists have many treatment plans to suit individual sufferers. Some researchers feel diet plays an important role in this systemic disease. Drugs can often control and contain the damage to joints and in some instances; the condition will stop with time. I have seen patients follow an anti-inflammatory diet, get psychological counseling, get more rest, get out of stressful relationships or job, take supplements and receive treatment to restore normal joint function of the spine and then start exercising. All of this combined stopped the autoimmune process in the few that actually took this advice. For most, the drugs are an easy, even if not, a permanent solution.

If your chronic backache/pain is of a dull, nagging, constant nature that gets worse at night but is relieved by aspirin, then you need to have blood tests to rule out an arthritide.

Surprisingly, systemic disorders are not limited to older people. For men, Ankylosing Spondylitis, a form of rheumatoid arthritis, can begin in the early twenties. The first sign of this condition is a dull back pain that gets worse with activity and becomes increasingly sharper. Later it is accompanied by severe fatigue, irritability, and increased pain after any aggressive physical or manipulative therapy.

This disease causes widespread inflammation of the spinal joints and starts in the sacroiliac, pelvic joints. No one is sure of the cause of Ankylosing Spondylitis, but it is characterized by the following: a flattening of the hollow of the lower back, a loss of forward and backward bending, severe stiffness in the spinal joints, and a constant, nagging, aching pain that only an anti-inflammatory can relieve.

This condition is very often mis-diagnosed in the early stages, which is a shame, because it has a specific blood marker easily detected by a simple blood test. Fortunately the progression of this crippling disease can be slowed considerably by anti-inflammatory drugs and daily exercise sessions on a stationary bicycle. Yes, the exercise will help if the patient is on the correct drugs.

Despite today's great technical advances in the healing arts, the incidence of arthritis in all its' varied forms, along with many other degenerative diseases, is not decreasing. Over the years there have been many studies showing that a less stressful environment, more physical exercise and natural foods can produce a population with less degenerative disease. Many factors contribute to the development of degenerative diseases; attending to as many as possible makes good sense. It always seemed odd to me that a person would take an anti-inflammatory drug with all its'side effects and not address the contributory causes of the inflammation.

Psychiatrists and clinical psychologists are rarely recommended for chronic degenerative back pain, yet they can be a big help in a number of stress-related cases. I have had the cooperation of many patients over the years, which have improved their eating habits and living patterns and thus stopped the progression of a degenerative disease.

Smoking uses up your supply of vitamin C as well as depleting your immune response by constantly inhaling toxins. The immune response can fatigue and not be able to fight cancer cells with the usual, normal virulence.

Birth control pills interfere with the utilization of the B vitamins. Both B and C are needed to heal inflammation. I can assure you that the average American diet is not healthy, and our backs suffer from the inadequate intake of essential macro and micro nutrients. Most people eat far too many saturated animal fats, refined sugars and carbohydrates and excesses of meat, at the expense of little or no raw fruits and vegetables. "We are what we eat", is not far from the truth. Our cells are constantly dying and being replaced so it is never too late to start eating healthily.

Healthy joints and discs need quality protein. We only need around 8 ounces a day. However, overcooking changes the protein so "rare" is better.

The back pain of anemia is also a nagging pain and accompanied by fatigue, a loss of energy and irritability. This again is easily confirmed by blood tests.

Osteoporosis/Pregnancy

More than 25% of all post-menopausal women suffer from osteoporosis. This condition causes the bones of the spine to become brittle and vulnerable to compression and fracture. Osteoporosis in older women has many causes and Osteoporosis is always undergoing research all around the world. Some bones are more vulnerable than others and the spine is a common area affected.

It is widely accepted that lowered levels of estrogen is the cause of osteoporosis. Yet in countries where women walk everywhere they go there is less loss of bone density. Conversely women on the UCLA swim team who spend many hours a week in suspension in water have the onset of bone loss in their early twenties.

This prompts me to suggest to women taking hormones that they also make sure they do some anti-gravitational exercise like walking and weight lifting.

Vitamin D is needed to digest and utilize Calcium from the diet. The avoidance of sunshine lowers our production of Vitamin D. Halibut liver oil capsules are small and an easy way to assure no D deficiency develops. Cod liver oil capsules are much larger and tend to repeat a few minutes after swallowing them. Calcium tablets should have Magnesium with them. Some say in a one to one ratio and others at two to one. Just don't take it alone and try to take it on going to bed. It absorbs well on an empty stomach.

Another cause of systemic back pain requiring a special approach is pregnancy. More than 50% of pregnant women will get back pain from their fifth month of pregnancy on. Twenty-five percent of these mothers-to-be suffer daily and most suffer on a weekly basis. Sixty-five percent of these women have severe back pain during labor.

Back pain is most likely if a pregnant woman has developed mechanical dysfunctions, before she becomes pregnant. The postural changes due to the added weight out front, magnifies the already established and most likely, silently, compensated, locomotor problems. The most common culprit is a blocked sacroiliac joint of the pelvis. The free sacroiliac joint becomes overstretched and inflamed as it tries to compensate to the pregnancy, postural changes and the other dysfunctional sacroiliac joint.

The catch-22 is that the unborn baby can be adversely affected if the pregnant woman takes drugs to relieve her pain. The good news is that a Swedish study showed that seven out of ten prenatal back pain sufferers received complete relief from manipulation alone, without using drugs.

I once attended a woman who had already started the birthing process and was experiencing excruciating, sacroiliac pain. I was able to release the locked sacroiliac joint and she went on to have her baby relatively pain free. The mid-wife involved had seen the same thing once before, which gave me the confidence to gap the joint so it could move. The fact that birthing mothers have a hormone relaxin present in their system meant that I could use a minimum of force to get the sacroiliac joint to move.

After the birthing process, the hormone relaxin gradually leaves the system and the pelvic and lower back ligaments lose their extra elasticity and tighten up. If the joints are not functioning properly as they tighten, postnatal back pain occurs.

Manipulation is often necessary during and after pregnancy. There is not even one recorded ill effect in the literature, not one. All women preparing to give birth should be checked by a chiropractor or osteopath for proper biomechanics of the pelvis and lower back. Normal, fully mobile sacroiliac joints make for easier engaging of the baby's head into the birthing canal during delivery.

Examining for pelvic mobility is simple and should be included in the obstetrician's prenatal procedure. It is ironic because during the 1940s and 1950s obstetricians did more sacroiliac research than did orthopedists. In those days the orthopedists believed the sacroiliac joints did not move. But chiropractors, osteopaths and obstetricians did, and they knew they moved quite freely.

Any women suffering from postpartum back or groin pain should see a chiropractor or osteopath who does manipulation. Both will examine for symphysis pubis joint instability which often occurs after birthing. This pelvic joint instability causes a very harsh sacroiliac pain along with pain of the normally painless and stable pubis joint. This condition is confirmed by x-ray of the pelvis with the patient standing with one foot on a block of wood and the other leg hanging down. An unstable symphysis pubis will separate and the normal joint will just tilt. I have seen many of these over the years, as it is overlooked by most doctors. Treatment for this complication of the birthing process requires the use of a trochanteric support belt 24 hours a day until the pain subsides.

A healthy person does not suffer from systemic disease. All systemic back disorders including gout and psoriasis are usually accompanied by changes in one's general health. Many cancers rear their ugly heads initially as back pain. These are characterized by tenderness and local pain which is constant and unaffected by rest or activity, and usually accompanied by fatigue and a loss of appetite. These cancers of the spine can be detected by bone-scan, or blood tests, and if caught in time can often be treated effectively. X-rays are only sensitive to 40% bone loss and CT scans detect 7% change. If you are experiencing a very localized pain in the bone and the x-ray is negative, insist on getting a scan. Early detection of disease is essential, if treatment is to be effective.

Incidents of back pain caused by Lyme disease are on the rise. Lyme disease is a disorder contracted from being bitten by a deer tick when out on a walk. The tick carries the disease organism that transmits to humans. It is not as unusual as it sounds because of the many wilderness and camping areas in America with deer populations. People visiting or living in these areas (especially the northeastern region) run the risk of being bitten and infected. If you discover a tick on you, go to a doctor immediately for antibiotics to prevent a horrible experience. It is easy to prevent and quite difficult to cure once it gets a hold on you.

There are many other less common systemic diseases. If your back pain is accompanied by a decline in your health, you should consult with your doctor as soon as possible. Systemic diseases should not be treated with home remedies; you need a doctor's supervision.

Stress-Induced Back Pain

Most specialists will agree that stress is a major contributor to many back disorders. Chronic stress causes a hormonal change in the body's chemistry. Worry, fear, hate, anger, frustration and pent-up emotions cause chemical reactions in the brain, triggering a chain of events that can result in muscle spasm and pain. The acute, severe pain of muscle spasm leads to more anxiety and stress, which in turn cause more muscle spasms, and more pain. It is all a vicious cycle.

I once treated and counseled a man who had never had a back pain in his life; until he arranged to see his 21-year-old daughter for the first time in 19 years. The day after he bought his airplane tickets, he began experiencing a terrible, shooting pain which doubled him over and almost completely immobilized him. Of course he missed his flight, but he did recover in a few weeks.

Then, three weeks later, on the day before he was to fly out again, he had his second disabling back attack. Apparently the man's guilt and fear about seeing his daughter caused a spill-over of tension into his lower back muscles. In Latin, soma refers to muscle. Some emotions are suppressed and express themselves in the soma and hence the term "psychosomatic back pain".

On many occasions, I have treated patients who experienced immediate reversal of the locked joint and muscle spasm. Upon feeling this painless release, the patient oftentimes will begin crying emotionally and uncontrollably for several minutes. And just as often, the patient will have no idea as to the origin of these released feelings. Psychologists call this the somatization of an emotion.

If you have experienced these effects after a chiropractic or osteopathic manipulation, you should seek counseling. Don't let the suppressed emotions become ulcers, colitis, cancer or even a heart attack. Stress can increase the effects of pre-existing systemic, mechanical or degenerative causes of back pain.

It is not difficult to recognize stress-related mechanical dysfunction. Stress sufferers frequently perspire too easily. They have cold hands and cold feet, are easily startled, fatigued but not sound sleepers, have indigestion and are often acutely aware of their heart beating. They are edgy and have poor concentration. They react to situations rather than respond thoughtfully. In other words they are completely distressed.

See diagram 2 (next page) which shows the cycle of stress, muscle spasm, joint dysfunction and mechanical disorders.

DISTRESS CYCLE

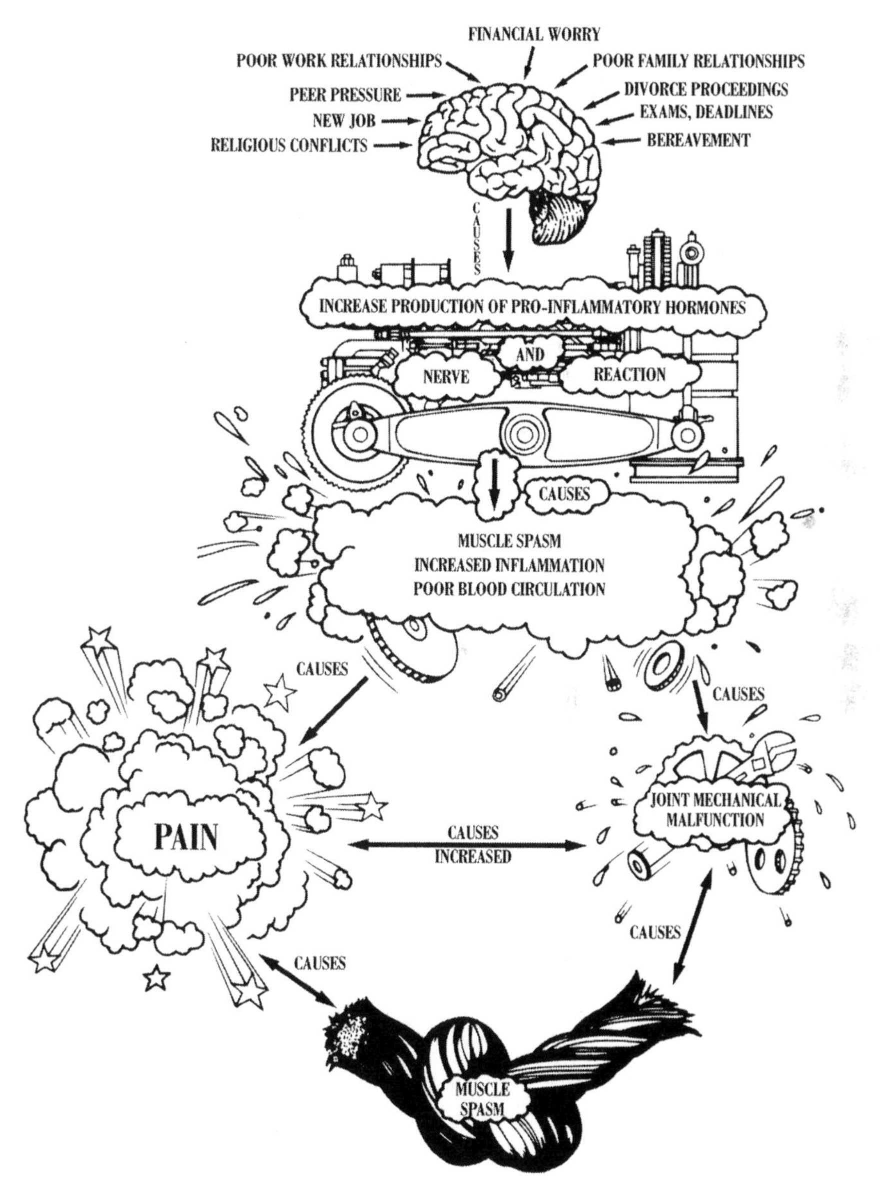

Diagram 2 Distress Cycle

In these pages you have read of many causes of back pain. In the next chapter you will identify which is the most likely cause or causes of your own back pain. In our next chapter, you also will be able to determine, through simple tests of a few questions, if you are one of the fortunate many, who after a few manipulations will be able to strengthen the core and other muscles. This is what we call the pro-active phase of treatment and can be done with low tech aids at home.

Chapter Two

"To be forewarned can set you free."

Faulty biomechanics and poor posture are the most common causes of back pain, and are the easiest to correct. This chapter will show you the difference between good and bad posture and normal versus abnormal mechanics.

The illustrations and tests included here will give you the opportunity to analyze yourself. You will be able to determine what type of back pain you have and evaluate your posture rating.

Taking the necessary steps to correct bad posture habits alone can alleviate some back pain. It can also save you the disappointment and financial losses of failed treatments. Chances are you're sitting incorrectly at this moment. Chances are, also, that your pour posture is a contributing factor to your back pain. The fact is, most people fall into a pattern of improperly sitting, standing and lying without even realizing that these activities are straining the back joints and shifting the weight from being evenly distributed between the discs and the back joints.

It is easy to fall into poor posture habits. Fortunately, by learning and using corrected biomechanics, it is quite possible to change these bad habits to good ones. The first step is the hardest. You have to become aware that these habits exist. To do that, you are going to have to be completely honest with yourself.

Do not downplay your symptoms.

A tough, hardy pig farmer once told me his back pain had started six months previously when he had bent over in a field. He had felt a sharp, sudden pain in the middle of one cheek of his buttock. The pain made him limp around for a few days, then it lessened to a constant dull ache. After six months he realized the pain wasn't going away, so he came to see if I could help him. To the amazement of both of us, an x-ray revealed the head of a bullet was suspended in his buttock muscles. That farmer was the ultimate sufferer. The original blood in his underwear was attributed to his hemorrhoids, and I guessed that some of his underwear was full of holes normally. A truly odd situation all caused by a careless rabbit hunter a few fields away.

After answering the following self-assessment questionnaire truthfully, you will discover your back pain more than likely has many causes. Some you can treat with self-help methods, while others will require that you see the appropriate back specialist for treatment.

Self-Assessment Quiz

This is one test you don't have to study for. So relax (hopefully sitting upright) and get ready to categorize your own particular back pain. Some of the questions require you to refer to specific photos or diagrams to try out positions. Other questions require that you satisfy both, or all, conditions of the question in order to answer YES.

1. Are you over 40 years of age and experiencing your first constant back pain which came on for no apparent reason?

YES NO

2. Do you have constant back pain that is only relieved by the use of aspirin or other arthritis pain killers?

   YES NO

3. Is your constant back pain or ache accompanied by the need to urinate often, more frequently than usual?

   YES NO

4. Is your back pain or ache accompanied by great fatigue, loss of appetite and or weight loss?

   YES NO

5. Ever since a certain incident, has your back pain radiated to your genitals and did they also become numb?

   YES NO

6. Ever since a certain incident, has your back pain become much more severe and does it radiate down your leg to your foot, accompanied by occasional or constant numbness?

   YES NO

7. Ever since a certain incident, has your back pain become worse and have you developed difficulty in urinating or becoming sexually aroused?

   YES NO

8. Do you have leg pain and notice your foot catches on the ground quite often?

   YES NO

9. If you have pain in one leg, try sitting down and raising the good leg and then the bad leg, straight out, parallel to the floor, as shown in Figures 1 and 2. Do you feel the pain increased in the bad leg, buttock or low back?

   YES NO

10. Is your back pain accompanied by swelling in the back or legs?

    YES NO

11. Has your back pain constantly persisted for more than one year?

    YES NO

12. Do you have pain in both legs at the same time?

    YES NO

13. Do you have numbness in either of your thighs?

    YES NO

14. Does pain in your back or leg start after you walk a certain distance and is it relieved by sitting, resting a short time?

    YES NO

15. Do you have great difficulty when trying to walk on your toes or heels?

    YES NO

16. Do you have severe leg pain without back pain?

    YES NO

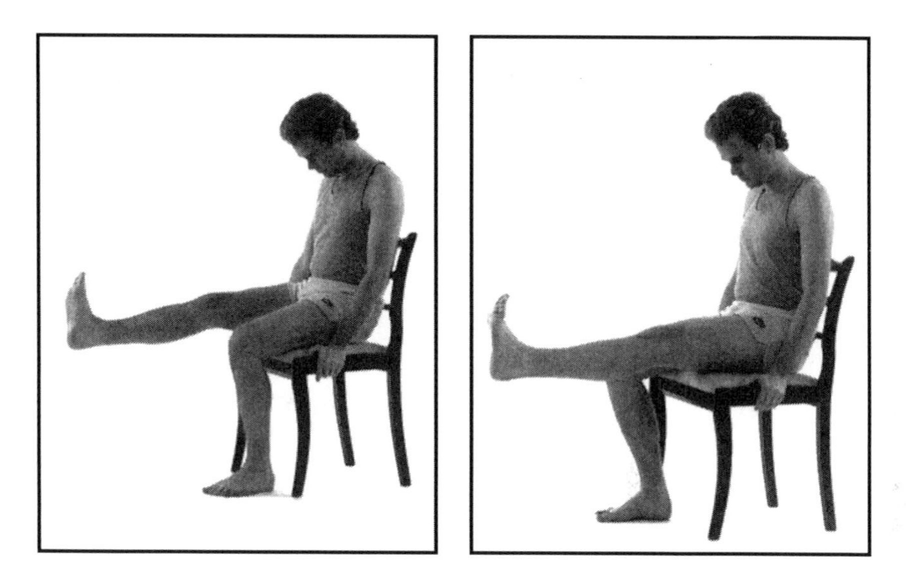

Fig. 1 and Fig. 2
This is a test for lumbar disc herniation. The right or left painful leg is resting, the knee bent with the foot flat on the floor. The pain-free leg is straightened. If attempting this maneuver causes back pain that increases when you nod your head forward, you need to see a chiropractor, osteopath or medical doctor.

If you answered YES to one or more of the questions in this group, it is important that you seek a doctor's opinion as soon as possible. You have a serious complication to one of the four groups of back pain (mechanical, degenerative, systemic, stress-induced). You'll need a prime contact doctor; a chiropractor, medical or osteopathic practitioner is the best place to start.

If you answered NO to all of the previous questions, then your next step is to take the following tests in order to determine your specific type of back pain. Once you know what you have, and what the contributing causes are, then you can sensibly select the correct professional advisor to stop that back pain for good. Remembering, none of their treatments are lasting if you don't follow up with the proactive home or gym workouts.

If you did answer NO to all the questions above, you are among the 90% of back pain sufferers who have mechanical disorders that cause reactive inflammation, muscle spasm and pain. These conditions are divided into the following groups:

1. Disc related
2. Back joint related
3. Sacroiliac joint related
4. Soft tissue related (muscles, tendons, ligaments, fascia)

Sometimes a sufferer has more than one area of inflammation and therefore is suffering from more than one condition at the same time. All these conditions improve quickly if caught early and can even be treated effectively with time if they have chronic changes. In order for you to determine which group you are in, it is necessary to answer the next group of questions. You could score less than the full number of points required for each diagnosis. However, most likely you will score high in one area. If you score high in more than one area, then you have more than one problem. This is not uncommon.

Test For Mechanical Group One: Disc Syndrome (Non-Herniated)

1. Does your back pain increase when you cough, sneeze or bend forward or if you bend your head forward, chin to chest?

   YES NO

2. Does sleeping relieve your back pain and/or leg pain, and after being up for a few minutes, does the pain return?

   YES NO

3. Does sitting increase back and /or leg pain?

   YES NO

4. When lying on your back on the floor, are you unable to raise your painful leg more than 15 inches off the ground? (See Figures 3, 4,and 5)

   YES NO

5. Lie face down with your shoulders raised and supported by a pillow for 15 minutes, as shown in Figure 6. Does the leg pain stop and the pain now center in the lower back?

   YES NO

6. When standing, are you forced to hunch forward and/or to one side?

   YES NO

7. Does your back pain radiate into your buttock on one side and go down the outside or back of your thigh?

   YES NO

8. Is the range of motion in your lower back greatly restricted or does your back lock up at certain, hitch points?

   YES NO

SCORING

Score 2 points for each YES answer to the previous questions. If you scored ten or more, you most likely have a lumbar disc syndrome. If you scored less or even if you scored more than ten please complete all the following questions as you may have more than one problem at the same time.

Test For Mechanical Group Two: Back Joint Syndrome

1. Is the pain in your back in a specific area and to one side or with some people radiating across both sides but close to the mid line.

   YES NO

2. Does the pain from your back radiate to the back of the thigh of one leg?

   YES NO

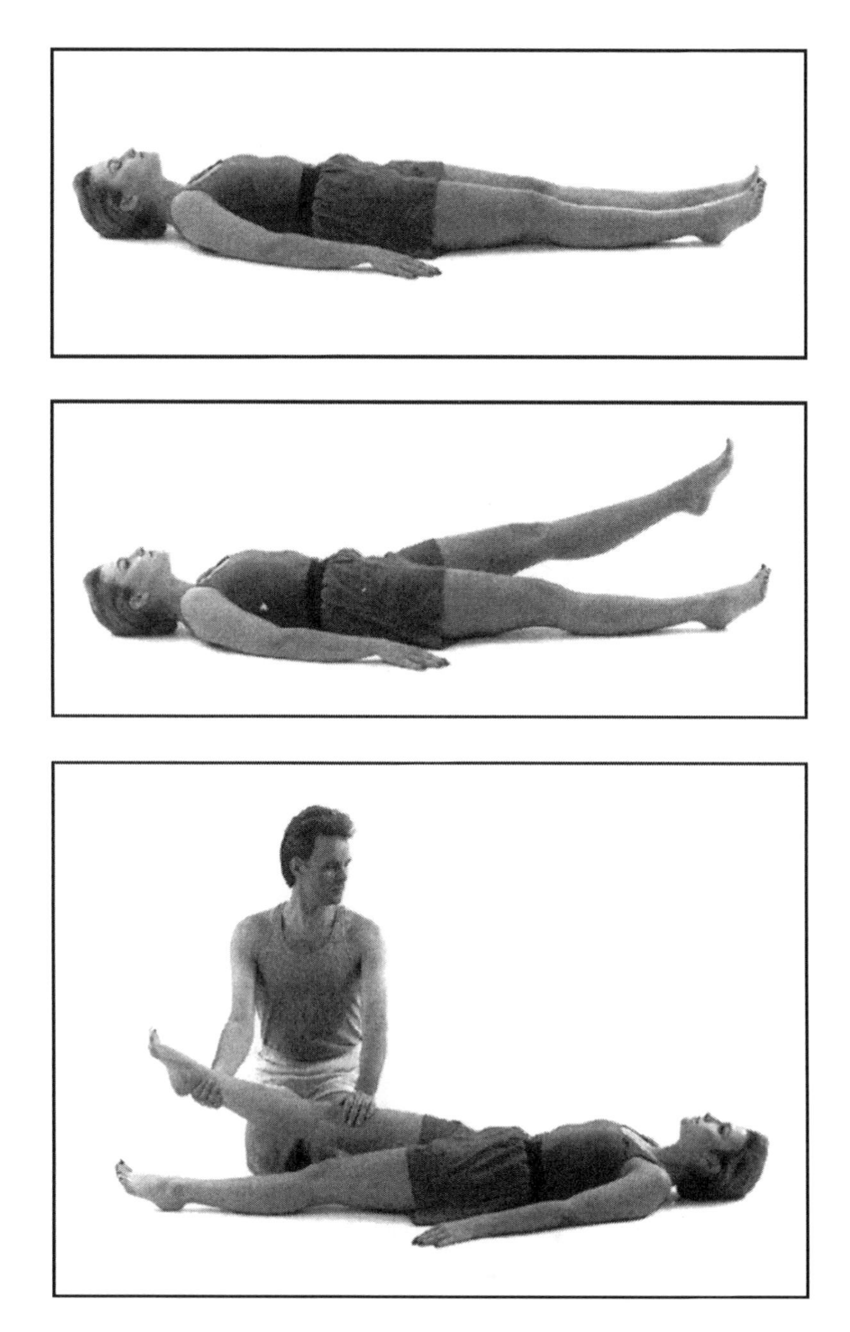

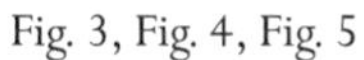
Fig. 3, Fig. 4, Fig. 5
When a disc has protruded, but not necessarily herniated or ruptured, neither the sufferer nor a friend can raise the painful leg past 20 degrees (about 15 inches) from the floor.

3. Can you ease the pain by bending slightly forward?

YES NO

4. Does the pain intensify if you bend backwards?

YES NO

5. Lie on your back as shown in Figures 7 and 8. Can you or a friend raise your leg off the floor to 75 degrees or more before you feel any pain?

YES NO

SCORING

Score two points for each YES answer to the previous group of questions. If you scored eight or more points, you most likely have an inflamed back joint.

Test For Mechanical Group Three: Sacroiliac Syndrome

1. Is the pain very low on one side of the lower back and does it radiate to the front groin, side and back of the thigh?

YES NO

2. Does your range of motion feel more restricted in the hip joint than in the back?

YES NO

3. While lying on your back as shown in Figures 9 and 10, do you feel pain when you or a friend raises your legs between 30 to 60 degrees off the floor?

YES NO

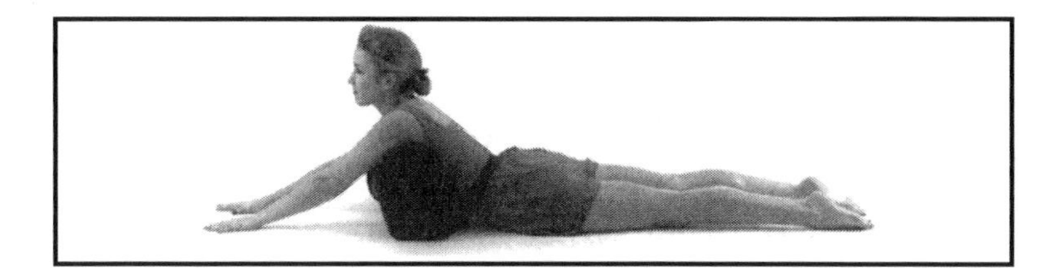

Fig. 6
A New Zealand physiotherapist discovered this test by accidentally leaving a back and leg pain sufferer in this posture for 15 minutes or so. The leg pain disappeared and centered more in the lower back. If you have leg pain, try it. If your leg pain moves towards your back and is less far down your leg after 15 minutes, rejoice! You should get better and stay better, with the suggestions in this book.

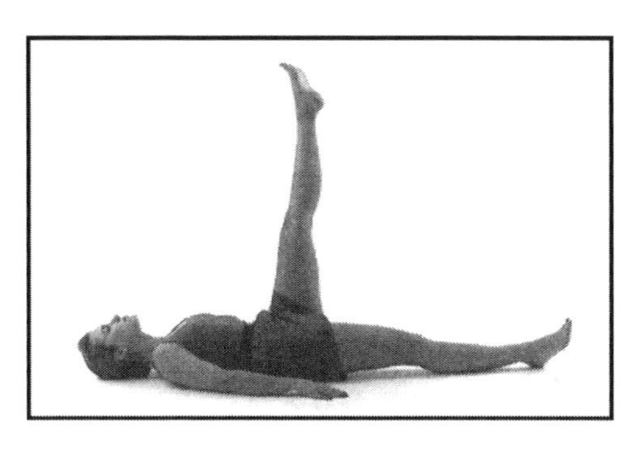

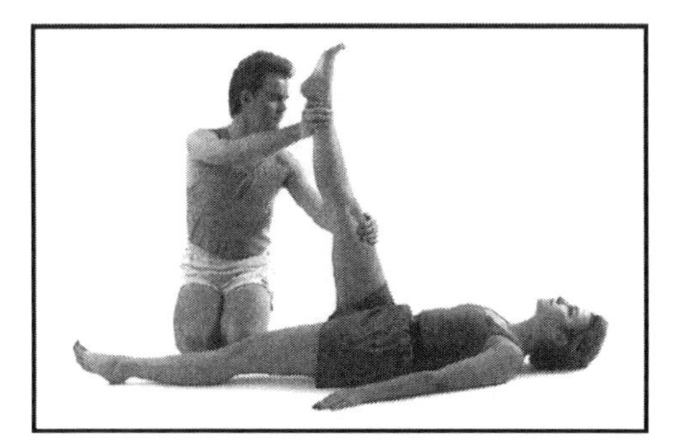

Fig. 7, Fig. 8
When you or a friend raise your leg to this height, the pelvis tips and flattens the hollow in your lower back. As this lower back movement occurs the inflamed back joint starts to feel painful. If raising the leg causes leg pain or a tight pull at the back of your leg, this test has uncovered other problems which will be discussed later.

4. Lying on your back as in Figure 11, bend your painful leg at the knee with the outside of the ankle crossed over the other straightened leg. Do you feel pain in the lower back when you push your bent leg towards the floor?

   YES NO

5. Upon wakening, is your back very stiff, causing you to get out of bed with difficulty, and then does your back loosen up and get better as the day goes on?

   YES NO

6. Do you have difficulty transitioning from the seated to the standing position; then does it eventually get easier as you walk

   YES NO

SCORING

Score 2 points for each YES answer to the previous group of questions. If you scored eight or more, you most likely have a sacroiliac joint problem.

Test For Mechanical Group Four: Muscle Syndrome

1. Does putting pressure on the deeper layer of muscles in the lower back refer the pain to the groin, back and front of the thigh?

   YES NO

2. When lying down, can you or a friend raise your legs one at a time to 90 degrees with no back pain?

   YES NO

3. By probing with care using your fingers, can you locate the muscle that hurts, and by pressing on a certain spot in the muscle for a few minutes, find relief?

   YES NO

SCORING

Score two points for each yes answer to the previous group of questions. If you scored four or more, you most likely have a muscle, trigger point problem.

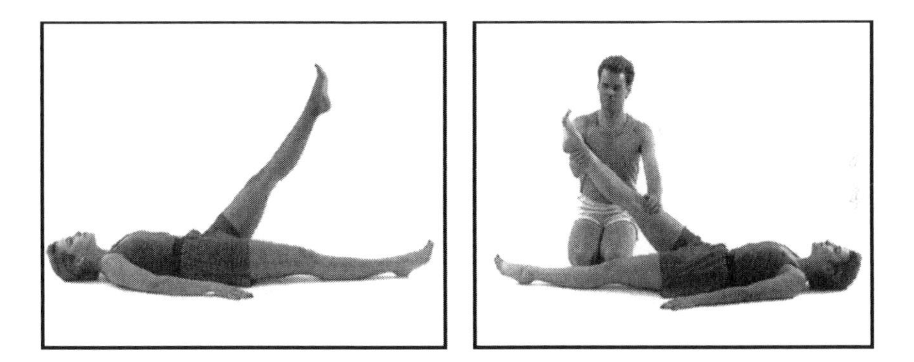

Fig. 9, Fig. 10
Raising your leg or having your leg raised to 60 degrees will cause sacroiliac joint pain. The back pain will occur before the lumbar spine flattens to the floor. The pain will be very low and to the side, almost to the hip joint.

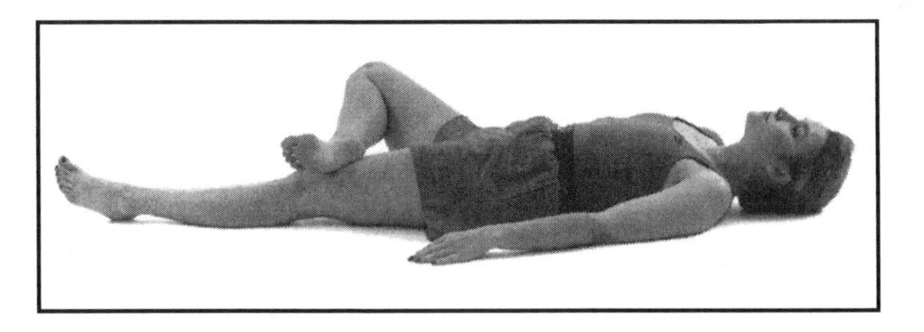

Fig. 11
Place the leg that's on the same side as your lower back pain across your straightened leg and form a figure four (4). If pressing your bent knee to the floor increases your lower back pain, it is most likely your sacroiliac joint is inflamed. If you can't do this test because your bent knee is stuck up in the air, you have a hip joint problem that is probably playing havoc with your lower back pain condition.

To repeat, you may have discovered through the above scoring that your back pain originates from more than one of the above conditions. This is not uncommon and each condition will need to be treated specifically by your chiropractor or other health practitioner. However, the home care exercises and stretches presented in this book will help the recovery from all the conditions, at one stage or another of the recovery process.

If you are one of the majority of back pain sufferers in the mechanical category, the next chapter will help you choose the correct practitioner, or be assured that your present practitioner is right for your causes of the pain.

However, before we move on you also need to assess your posture and muscle/joint flexibility. Lack of good posture and/or poor muscle/joint flexibility will adversely affect your ability to achieve lasting results in the treatment of your back pain. Once again, you must answer YES or NO. A NO reply here will mean poor posture or loss of flexibility is involved in your back problem, even if a lifting incident initiated the first pain.

Posture, Muscle/Joint Tests

1. When looking at yourself in a full length mirror, do your shoulders and hips appear to be level?

   YES NO

2. While standing in a relaxed manner, as shown in Figures 12 and 13, can you raise up onto your toes without rocking forward? (Figure 13 is normal.)

   YES NO

3. Refer to Figures 14, 15 and 16. Can you sit on your heels (squat) with your feet parallel and twelve inches apart while leaving your heels on the ground? (Figures 14 and 15 are normal; Figure 16 is incorrect.)

   YES NO

4. While standing with your feet slightly apart and parallel, can you lean backward without twisting, and touch the back of each knee?

   YES NO

5. While standing with your feet slightly apart and parallel, can you lean forward with straight legs and touch your toes?

   YES NO

6. While standing with your feet slightly apart and parallel, can you lean to each side without twisting and reach to the outside of each knee?

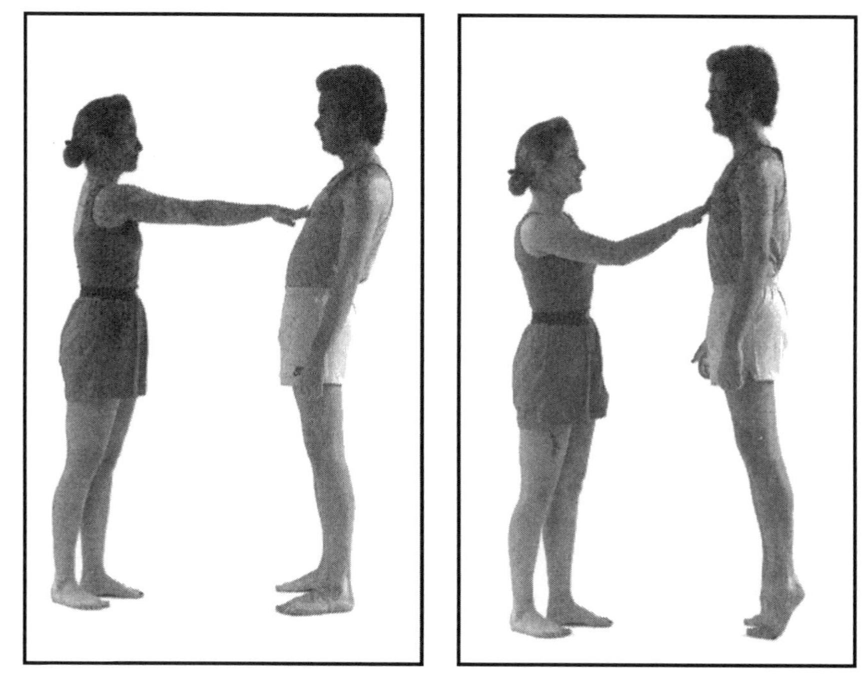

Fig. 12 Fig. 13

Ninety percent of back pain sufferers stand with too much weight on the back joints instead of forward onto the discs where the weight belongs. To test if this is one of your problems, have someone lightly place a finger on your chest bone. If you have to rock forward a few inches before you can raise up onto your toes (Figure 12), you have this bad posture problem. Good posture is standing at the point where you can raise up onto your toes without rocking forward, as in Figure13.

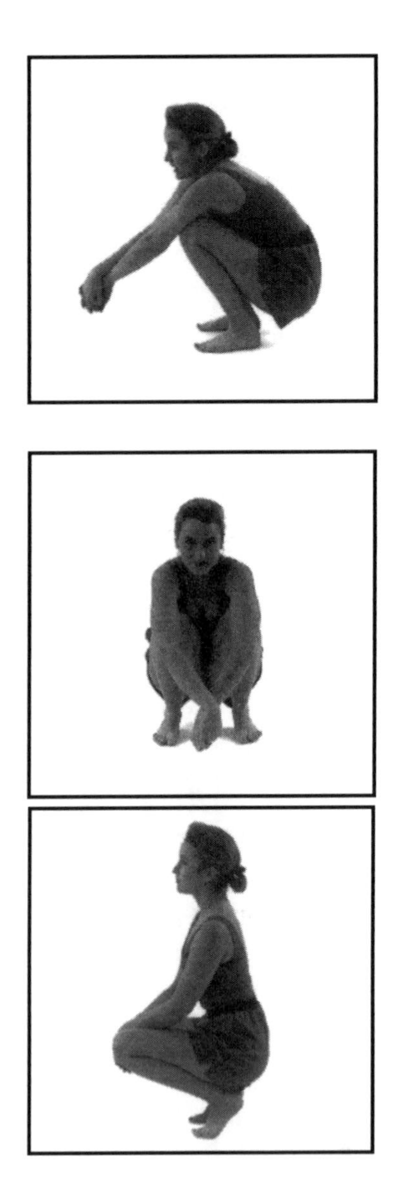

Fig. 14, Fig. 15, Fig. 16
In countries where people squat as in Figures 14 and 15, there is much less degenerative disc disease at the age of 55. If your flexibility is not good enough, you will squat incorrectly, as shown in Figure 16. Learn to squat correctly by holding onto a counter top or sink front, making sure your heels stay flat on the floor. This stretch is a real winner. Persist until you can comfortably squat this way for a few minutes.

7. When lying on your back with your hip flexed at 90 degrees and your other leg lying on the floor, can you then straighten your bent leg so that it is perpendicular to the floor? See Figures 17, 18 and 19; figure 18 shows how the leg should straighten.

   YES NO

8. While lying on your back, can you pull one knee to your chest while your straight leg remains flat on the floor? Refer to Figures 20 and 21 for an illustration. Figure 20 shows that the leg should not bend at the knee.

   YES NO

9. When lying face down, can you bend your knee, and pull it in so that your heel is touching your buttock? See Figures 22, 23 and 24.

   YES NO

10. Lying face down as shown in Figure 25, can you lift your arms and legs off the floor at the same time?

    YES NO

11. Lying face up, can you do a a knees-bent sit-up without anchoring your feet? See Figure 26

    YES NO

12. Lying on your side with your feet anchored, can you raise your shoulders 10 to 12 inches off the floor? Figure 27 correctly demonstrates this diagnostic exercise.

    YES NO

13. Sit on the floor with the bottoms of your feet together as shown in Figure 28. Can you easily bring your knees close to the floor?

    YES NO

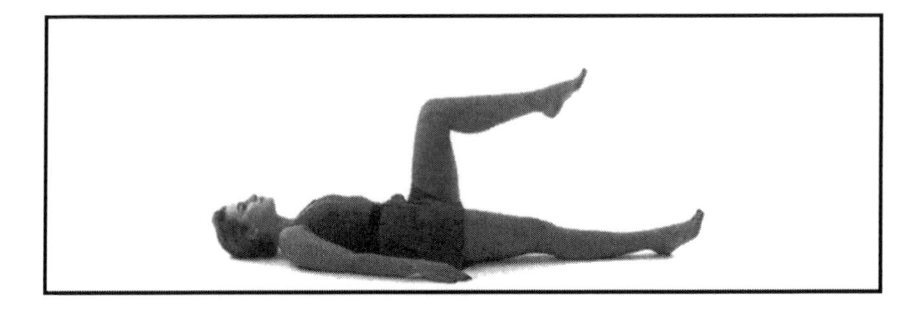

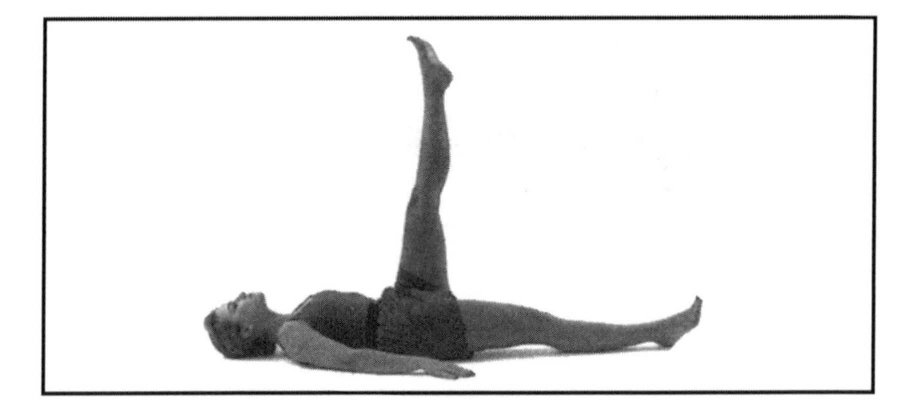

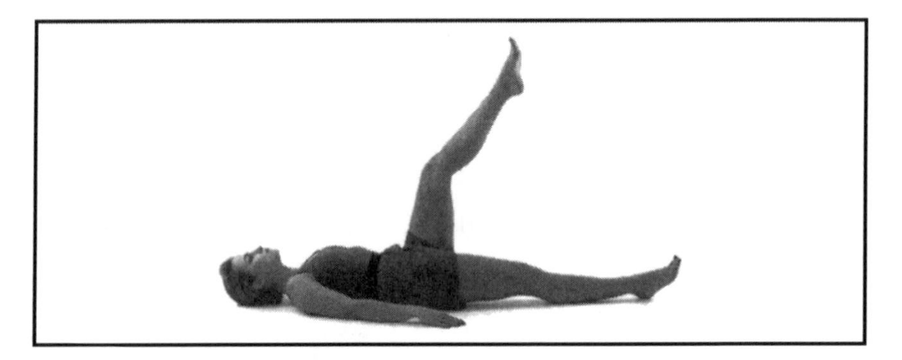

Fig. 17, Fig. 18, Fig. 19

The hamstring muscles at the back of your thigh should be long enough to allow you to straighten your leg from the position in Figure 17 to the position in Figure 18. If your leg does not straighten, guesstimate the number of degrees short of straightening. The bigger the angle away from a straight leg the shorter the hamstrings. The shorter your hamstrings, the more likely it is that they are affecting your back pain. It is tantamount to malpractice to be treated for a bad back and not be getting help for short hamstrings!

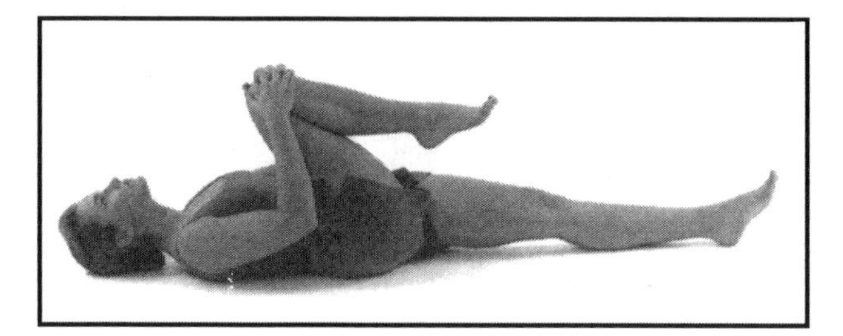

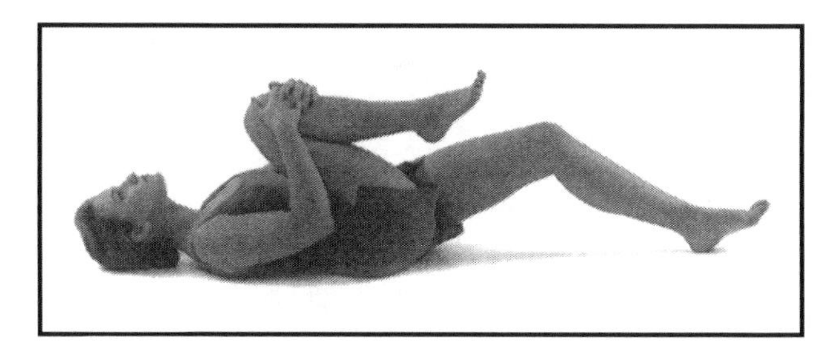

Fig. 20, Fig. 21
The large and very powerful hip flexor muscle (psoas muscle, pronounced SO-AS) anchors to your lower back vertebrae and becomes a major factor in faulty lower back mechanics. If the psoas muscle is too short, you cannot keep the opposite leg relaxed and extended flat on the floor, while you pull one knee towards your chest.

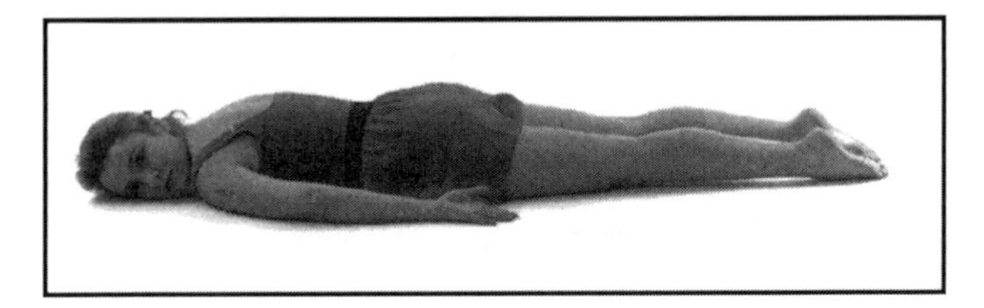

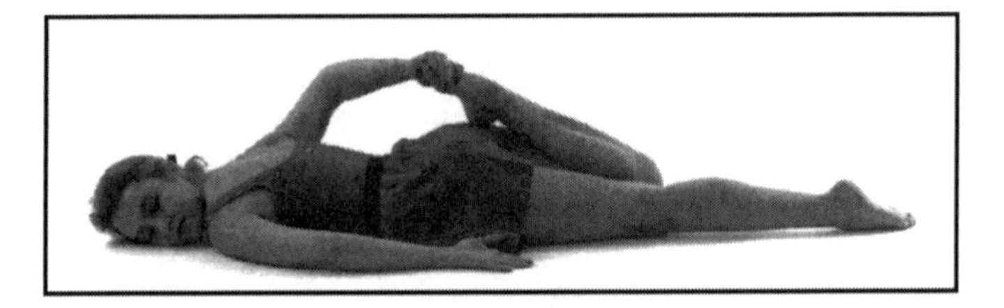

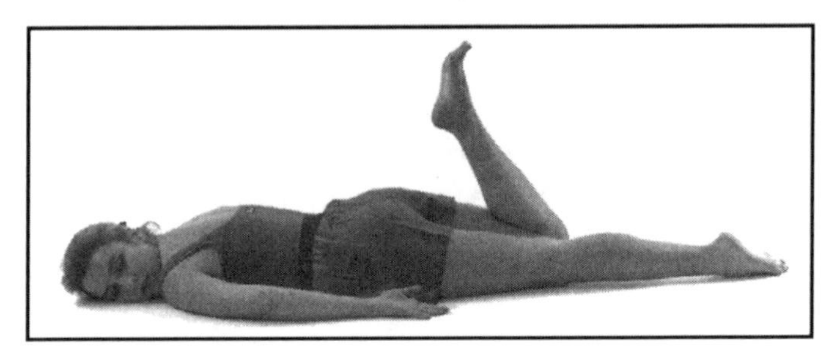

Fig. 22, Fig. 23, Fig. 24
The large quadriceps muscles (called "quads") that form the front of your thigh should be long enough to allow you to easily place you heel on your buttock while lying face down. The shorter your quads, the further your heel will be from your buttock and the more likely it will be that this is a part of your lower back problem.

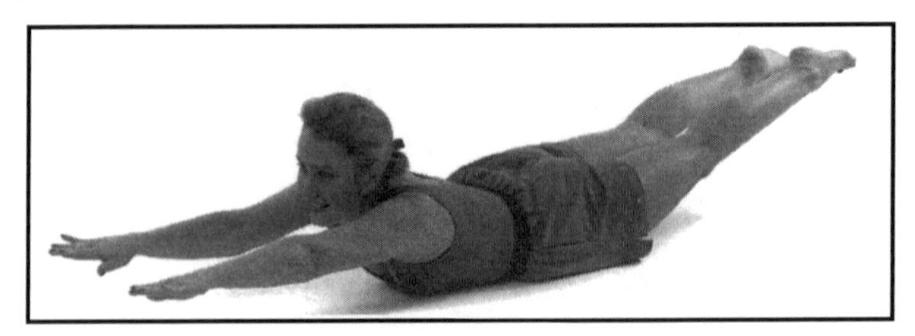

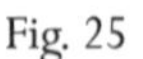

Fig. 25
In chronic lower back pain sufferers, the extension muscles are weak. You should be able to easily hold your hands and feet in the air at the same time for a count of 10. You will need electric muscle stimulation to tone these muscles if your back is painful and inflamed. If this exercise does not produce a lingering pain, you can commence our recommended extension exercises.

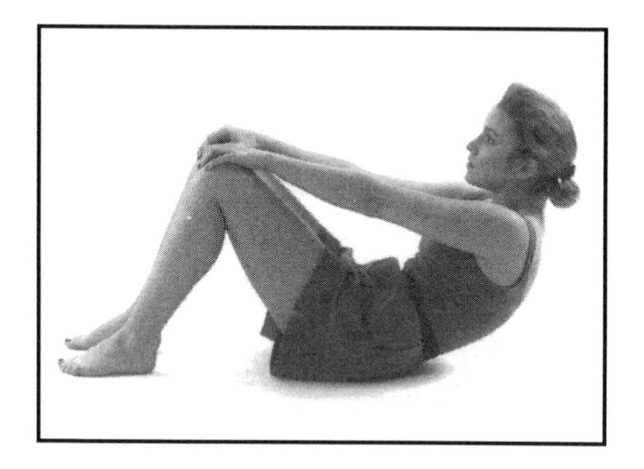

Fig. 26
Because your back is hurting, test the strength of your abdominal muscles with a gentle sit-up. Hold the above sit-up for 10 seconds and then let yourself down to the floor slowly. If you can't hold your rib cage off the floor without using your arms or anchoring your feet, you need to considerably strengthen your abdominal muscles.

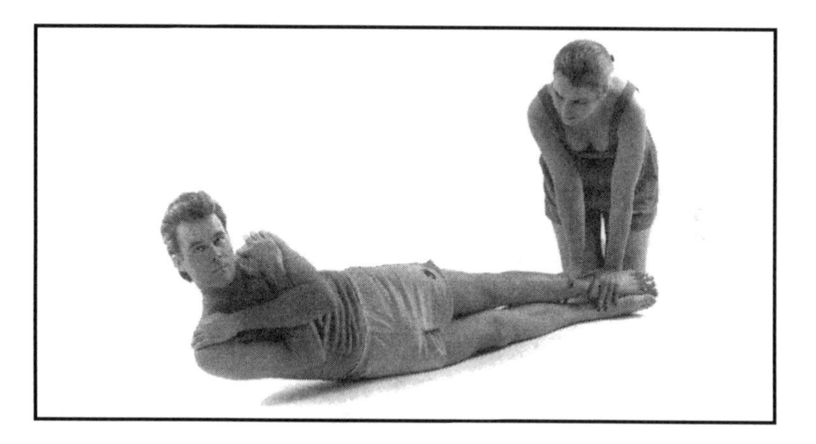

Fig. 27
The most important muscle stabilizer for the lower back is the lateral bending muscle called the quadratus lumborum, or QL muscle. Chronic back pain sufferers rarely have strong QL muscles. Before you try to lift yourself up sideways, make sure your upper shoulder does not rotate backwards. This cheating action will use the abdominals. Some famous athletes I have treated for chronic back pain could not do this exercise. You should be able to lift your bottom shoulder 10-12 inches off the floor.

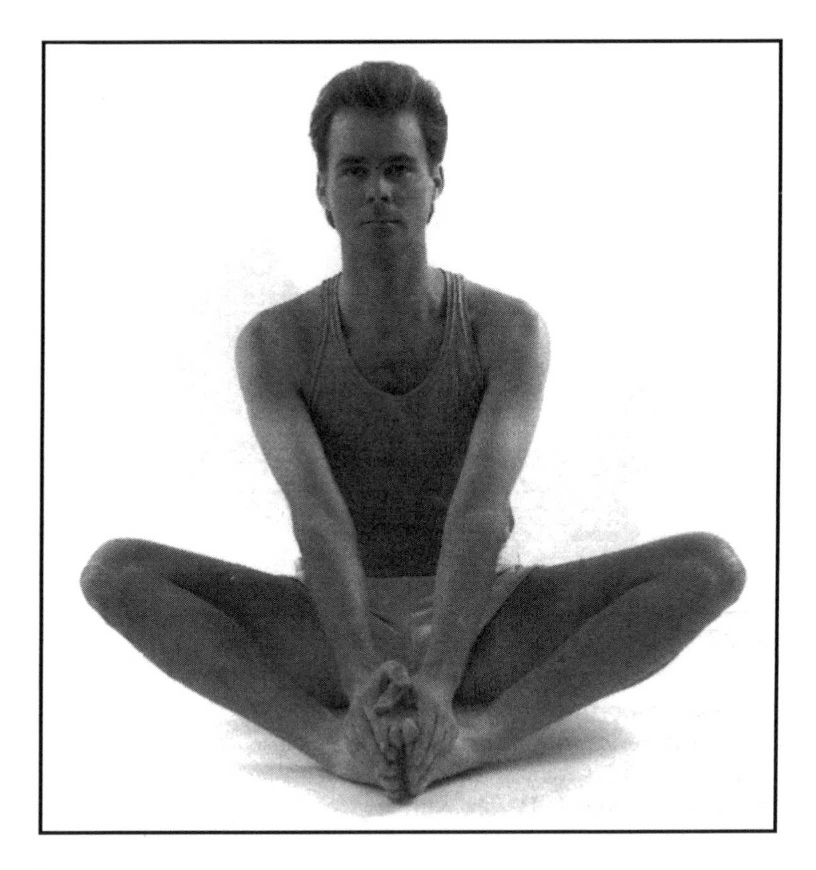

Fig. 28
This posture determines if your hip joints are flexible enough to have a pain-free back. If you cannot bring one or both knees close to the floor, either the groin muscles are too short or your hip joint is restricted. A doctor will need to determine whether one or both is the case. The good news is that you can change the range of motion in both cases. The bad news is that it takes perseverance over many months, often with professional help. Difficulty with this position reveals a significant finding. Don't ignore it!

14. Stand straight at ease. Look down at your ankles. Are the two bands of Achilles tendons perpendicular to the floor?

YES NO

15. Take a look at your knee caps. Are they pointing forward like the headlights of a car?

YES NO

16. Step down from a step. Do you need to rotate the foot on the step outward in order to lower the swinging foot down one step.

YES NO

SCORING

A NO answer to any of the previous group of questions indicates you have a posture problem or shortened and/or weakened muscles. Not correcting these faults is foolish. These are the problems that cause the recurrence of back pain before the degenerative changes occur. Chapter five describes how you can work and play to correct them.

Pain may be the reason you cannot easily perform some of these actions. If you are presently under professional care, and you are not working at correcting these shortened muscles and restricted joints, it is highly unlikely you will be able to stop your back pain for very long. You probably will continue to experience episodes of acute pain or attacks until a surgical crisis occurs or old age solves the problem with a natural fusion of the bones.

Look at the following posture diagrams. These will enable you to see how you compare to desirable postures. Having a friend help you would be useful, but a full length mirror will also do the job.

Turn sideways, stand in your usual posture. If your belly is flat, you are in good shape most likely. If your stomach protrudes but your back is only slightly curved forward with a little hollow you are not that bad. However, if you have a "pot belly" and an exaggerated hollow in the lower area of your back, then you're in trouble.

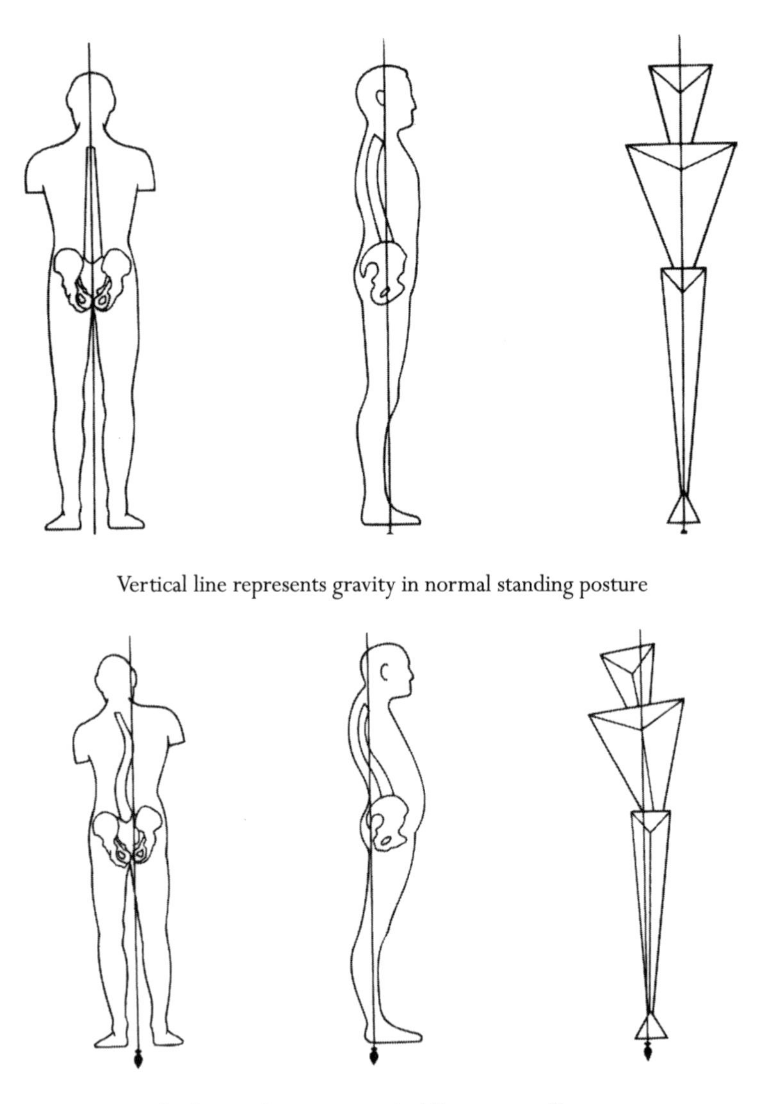

Vertical line represents gravity in normal standing posture

In abnormal posture, vertical line moves off center

Now look at your head. If it is being carried high above the shoulders, that's great. Your head should not be hanging low in front of your shoulders. Poor head/neck posture causes stress in the lower back region, further complicating the recover process.

At this juncture you should be able to identify the cause or causes of your back pain. If you are still not sure, go back and review the first two chapters. Take the next step in selecting the correct professional only after you are certain of the cause or causes of your ailment.

Diagnosis Summary

Non-Mechanical and Severe Disc Syndrome:

If you answered YES to one or more of the questions from the first group of questions on pages 36-37, you must go to a chiropractic, medical or osteopathic doctor. You need to be sent for screening tests such as X-rays, MRI, CT scan and lab work.

Mechanical Conditions and Their Symptoms

1. DISC SYNDROME
   Back and leg pains get worse as the day progresses. Your back locks up at certain points. Flexing your neck forward and coughing at the same time hurts in your low back. You can't raise your legs off the ground while they are out straight.

2. BACK JOINT SYNDROME
   The back pain is over a specific spot and usually to one side only. The pain eases when you bend slightly forward. Bending backward to one side increases the pain, which also may radiate to the back of the thigh on the same side.

3. SACROILIAC SYNDROME
   The pain is very low to one side of the lower back and radiates to the front, side and back of the thigh. The pain at the front is in the groin area and often patients feel it is in their hip. You wake up almost unable to get out of bed. Then as the day goes on, and you struggle to get around, the pain eases considerably until you try to lift something.

4. MUSCLE SYNDROME
   You can dig around with your thumb and find the exact spot that causes you pain and it radiates pain when you press on it. Continued deep pressure gives relief in a minute or so. This is called a Trigger Point. Muscle sprains and strains rarely occur, because we are hanging on our ligaments when we bend over to lift; especially if we lift with straight legs and not bending our knees.

Chapter Three

The Professionals

**"Admire the person who seeks the truth.
Beware of the person who has found it."**

Finding the right professional or specialist to treat your particular back pain is the single most important thing you can do to successfully overcome your problem. This chapter explains what the many different specialists offer. By understanding the orientation of each specialist, you will be able to find the proper practitioner to help you with your particular ailment. You will need to be in control of your own treatment plan under the guidance of a health professional.

Family Practitioner/Internist

Most people with minor back problems first seek the help of the family doctor. Whether they receive the proper care is highly speculative. A family practitioner or internist may be able to provide pain killers for temporary relief, but solving your problem is a low priority in his busy schedule back and forwards from the hospital. However, a responsible doctor should be able to recognize the different classifications of back ailments and refer you to the proper specialist.

Most family physicians are able professionals, but they are rarely back ailment specialists. You wouldn't think of going to your family doctor for a prescription for new glasses or Lasik eye surgery. Of course, you'd seek the advice of an ophthalmologist or optometrist. The same thing applies for those suffering from back problems. There are so many causes of back pain that it takes someone who is dealing with it daily to understand all the ramifications of the diagnosis and treatment. These specialists need the support of radiologists, oncologists, manual therapists and psychologists to mention a few. Normally pills only mask the effects of the persistent back pain and do not treat the underlying causes. Prescribing medication without treating the cause of the pain is tantamount to turning off the fire alarm and then leaving the scene of the fire.

The following questions/comments should be discussed and/or answered by your family practitioner who is looking after your back pain. To become an informed consumer of his healthcare ask the following questions, politely:

1. Have enough tests been ordered to determine whether the back pain is systemic or mechanical?
2. What is the diagnosis? Check this against the questionnaire in the previous chapter. (Does this make sense to you?)
3. Is the cause being treated, or are you receiving painkillers to suppress the symptoms?
4. If you are not getting the cause treated, ask for a referral to a recommended specialist. The specialist should deal with correcting the causes. (See further ahead in this chapter

for comments on chiropractors, orthopedists, osteopaths and physiotherapists, etc.)

5. Does your family doctor immediately refer you to an orthopedist? If you know you have mechanical back pain which is not an operative disc problem, do not waste your time and money seeing a surgical specialist. Manipulation of the locked joints, anti-inflammatory treatment of the inflamed tissues and stretching of the shortened muscles and ligaments, followed by strengthening exercises is the regimen of choice. These conservative methods are the norm for many modern doctors of chiropractic, who have made a paradigm shift from the old "misalignment" theories.
6. Does your family practitioner or internist object to the idea of Manipulation? If he or she is unaware of recent research studies conducted in the U.S.A., Canada, England and a few non-English speaking countries, which show the value of manipulation, it is time to take matters into your own hands and change doctors. Without changing the mechanical function the episodes will keep recurring.

Let's look at all the different specialists that accept back pain patients and see what they have to offer.

Orthopedist/Orthopedic Surgeon

The role of the orthopedist is to determine whether or not the patient is a candidate for surgery, or whether he or she should be referred to a physical therapist that rarely does manipulation.

It is a well known fact that back surgery leads the list of unnecessary surgical procedures. Canadian research indicated that only three per cent of chronic back pain sufferers actually need surgery! The other ninety seven percent can be managed with other more conservative methods. In the early 90s, research done in San Francisco indicated that only ten percent of the 240,000 back surgeries done in the USA every year, were necessary. Today, with the advent of mini surgeries that are much less invasive that number has risen greatly. Patients should be aware that a doctor specializing in surgery is more likely to treat the ailment surgically than in any other way. Always get a second opinion and ask which surgeons are more likely not to recommend a conservative approach.

Be very cognizant of this time factor: six months is a prudent waiting period from the onset of severe symptoms to actual surgery. However, there are situations when surgery should be done quickly. Watch your pain! If it is excruciating and persistent without let up, if there is substantial loss of reflex action or muscle weakness; if there is numbness or impairment of bodily functions like urinating or defecating; then surgery is necessary and should be done without delay. This surgical emergency is called the Cauda Equina Syndrome and waiting even 12 hours is too long. It is characterized by numbness in the private parts, severe excruciating pain trying to move and urine retention. I have only seen two cases in 47 years in practice, so it is not very common. However, failure to get surgical relief of pressure on the autonomic nerves will cause impotency and incontinency. Hospital emergency wards have been known to delay too long. Be very persistent if your disc syndrome degrades to this condition in a few hours. Don't wait to contact your practitioner, go to the emergency ward immediately; in an ambulance if you can't walk.

If you have already had unsuccessful surgery for a bad back, you have joined a large group of people in the failed, back surgery, syndrome classification. Many of these people have a sacroiliac or facet syndrome. The changes that showed on a MRI were actually a "red herring" and not the cause of the symptoms. The degenerative changes were present but the tests would not have co-related with disc syndrome. This lack of co-relation between MRI findings with the actual clinical picture is often ignored, because the patient is in severe pain and more than willing to undergo surgery. Forty percent of 40 year olds, who have no back symptoms, have arthritis and disc herniation according to published studies. Faulty mechanics leads to pathology but the pathological changes don't always lead to pain.

Of course a few failed back surgeries result from a surgeon error or poor healing with too many adhesions. However, after surgery, it is extremely important to make sure the mechanical causes are attended to, so that the surgical repair is not put under the same harmful stresses which caused the need for surgery. Far too often, a second and third surgery is needed the next levels up the lumbar spine, not too many years later.

Surgery is usually but not always needed when the soft center of the disc is extruded outside. It is like tooth paste being squeezed from the tube; it can't all be sucked back in.

The surgeon needs to go in and remove it and remove any spurs or adhesions causing compression of the nerves. Surgery is also needed if the spinal joints become very unstable and aberrant joint movement occurs that does not respond to conservative procedures. To detect instability, x-rays need to be taken with you bending forward and then backward to demonstrate the instability. If you are over fifty and your back pain does not respond to anybody's treatment and rehabilitation then insist on these x-ray, functional studies. Instability defies most conservative care. Most back surgery today involves a lot less invasive procedures and much quicker, recovery times.

I am pleased to say, in the last two years, back surgery has become far less radical, and fusions and laminectomies are not routine, anymore.

Neurologists

The nerve specialist will determine whether there is damage occurring to the nerves, which causes muscle wasting, muscle weakness and numbness in the extremities. It often happens that by the time the neurologist is consulted, surgery is already inevitable. The disc herniation, like a space-occupying tumor, must be removed. Yet, it is my experience that many borderline cases are less likely to be sent to a surgeon by a neurologist as the mild cases can often recover on their own. Nerves are as fluid and supple as mercury, it is not easy to trap and compress them, as is imagined.

There is some controversy in medicine as to whether a neurosurgeon or a orthopedic surgeon should do spinal surgery. It is my opinion that you need to do your due diligence to find a surgeon that doctors recognize as a "fine surgeon". He or she can be an orthopedic or a neurosurgeon. Your chiropractor or general practitioner will know who is best in your area or the hospital near you. Getting a second opinion is never a bad idea. Remember there is no hurry unless you are unable to urinate and have saddle numbness. A few extra days will not cause any permanent damage.

Do not get railroaded into unnecessary surgery. Small disc bulges as seen on M.R.I. and C.T. scan are also present in patients over 50 who never have back pain. If your doctor doesn't like the suggestion of your getting a second opinion, then switch doctors. Be wary of back surgery; it has a significant failure rate, when followed up a year later.

Scientific reports on surgery lack a control group of similar patients that did not undergo surgery. Thus surgeons report their observations in prospective studies, but they are not compared to a control group and certain conclusions they make, are really not qualified. One Italian study attempted this comparison and reported at the end of a year the two groups had similar outcomes. The surgical group had better, early relief and the non-surgical group was a little better, overall. The failure rates were about the same.

The Physiotherapists/Physical Therapists

These specialists have changed considerably in the last few years. They used to abhor manipulation and only work under the guidance and prescription of a medical doctor. In some of the states of America, they can now legally see patients, without a medical prescription. They have added a few years to their training, for those that wish to learn manipulation skills. I find, I can now co-treat with my local physiotherapists who don't manipulate. These patients we co-treat often tell me, "it is about time". A large portion of physiotherapists work in hospitals and specialize in all kinds of post-operative rehabilitation. The physiotherapists that deal with back pain are orthopedic physiotherapists and specialize in orthopedic, post-operative rehabilitation.

If you see or are going to see a physiotherapist as a prime contact doctor then be sure you are given a thorough examination. Remember ten percent of back pain conditions are systemic. Ask if these have been ruled out in the diagnostic work-up.

For your own protection, not to mention peace of mind, here is a list of questions that you need to ask your physiotherapist to see if the proper decisions are being made:

1. Have the appropriate tests been completed to diagnose my type of back pain? What is my working diagnosis?
2. Does my back pain have a systemic cause? If the answer is yes, you should also be under the care of a specialist that is prescribing and overseeing your care.
3. If you have mechanical causes of back pain, what are they?
   -Locked back joints?
   -Shortened muscle groups?
   -Locked sacroiliac joints?
   -Decreased hip function, range of motion?
   -Pronated ankle (collapsing inward)?
   -Poor posture, standing and sitting?
   -Improper muscle recruitment order?
4. Is my treatment getting at the causes of my pain as well as reducing the inflammation?
5. How are these underlying causes being monitored?
6. Why am I getting heat for inflammation? It may feel good at the time but it encourages swelling. Ice is better for any injury.
7. Can I get Electrotherapy or Low Level Infra Red Laser Therapy to reduce inflammation in your office and then use ice packs at home?

If you discover that the goal of your treatment is just relieving the pain and not treating the underlying causes, change your therapist. Otherwise you will only get temporary relief. Chiropractors and physiotherapists are beginning to realize, they need to merge their approach to your problem. Manipulation to restore joint function needs to be followed by exercise and stretching, and exercising and stretching needs to be preceded by restoring joint dysfunction. Find a physiotherapist who understands this relationship. There are a lot more around than you think. Heat and exercise may relieve your pain, but in the majority of cases, will not correct the cause of your back pain. If your prescribed physiotherapy is a class of ten, at a hospital, you are probably wasting your time. It takes a one on one ratio to get this job done.

Rheumatologists

Rheumatoid Arthritis is the single largest crippling disease in America, and one of the chief culprits of chronic joint pain. Rheumatologists specialize in the diagnosis and treatment of all the different forms of arthritis. There are many specific blood tests and imaging labs that help them arrive at a diagnosis. If you have a high score in the systemic cause of back pain, section of questions; you need to get these tests completed. If your pains do not respond to mechanical means or even cause a painful reaction each time over a reasonable period of time; it is time to see a rheumatologist.

For example a condition called Ankylosing Spondylitis, described in Chapter One, is often missed or misdiagnosed when it causes back pain in early adulthood. When these young adults do not improve with most treatments, good back specialists should recognize the need for a rheumatologists' opinion. In turn, a good rheumatologist should recognize the high incidence of psychological factors in a rheumatoid patient. Clinical psychologists should also be consulted to determine the cause of the harmful distress in these patients.

Painful muscle conditions called Fibrositis or Fibromyalgia can be confirmed by a Rheumatologist. These are very complex conditions to treat. Many mavericks make unsupported claims and these patients often run around from pillar to post with some success but rarely a complete solution. Some do well to manage this condition with dietary changes and supplements. A Paleolithic diet free of any grains has been shown to reduce inflammation. The supplementation with Ribose has given many, more energy, as it helps with the ATP replenishment in the muscle cells. Some get good relief from injection of the Trigger Points, in the many muscles involved in Fibromyalgia.

The truth is that so far nobody really knows why so many muscles in the body can pain at one time and also cause so much fatigue. It has been shown that sleep loss is linked to this condition.

In summary, if you get short term pain relief from aspirin or some other pain reliever, and/or your condition continually worsens, if treated by any of the manual therapies, you probably need to see a rheumatologist.

Chiropractors

Back pain conditions are the most common complaints seen in a chiropractors office, neck/shoulder pain is the second most common.

Manipulation is the main therapy supported by physical therapy and followed by rehabilitation.

For descriptive purposes, chiropractors often tell their patients the cause of back pain is spinal misalignment. They talk about bones being "out" and the nerves being "pinched". These are misnomers, as is the term "slipped disc". Discs rarely slip and most back pain is not caused by a bone being out of place. A nerve that is truly "pinched" causes pain down the arm or leg when accompanied by inflammation of that nerve. The fact is manipulation (the chiropractic adjustment) changes the mechanics of the joints and with repetition, establishes correct nerve, muscle and joint function.

Chiropractors deal with the mechanical group of back disorders, and refer bone cancer and other systemic conditions to other specialists. If you answered YES to one of the questions in the first diagnostic group, you could go to a chiropractor, but most likely you would be referred to another specialist after the diagnostic work-up. On the other hand, if you are suffering from a disc, back joint, sacroiliac joint, muscular or postural related back pain, you will be given a treatment schedule.

Research has shown that a very small percent of disc cases actually need surgery. Two separate studies comparing chiropractic manipulation to hospital outpatient treatment confirmed chiropractic procedures are safe and most effective for non surgical back conditions.

Chiropractic is going through a paradigm shift and it is estimated that fifty percent of today's practitioners, work to a functional model and fifty percent are still trying to realign the vertebra. The good news is that whatever the intention, the manipulations are similar. Those into restoring function tend to be more likely to specifically treat the inflammation and prescribe rehabilitation stretches and exercises.

The chiropractors, who have shifted to the more modern paradigm, understand the relationship between the lower extremity joints and spinal function. The locomotor system is a co-related chain, all reliant on each other, in order that we can perform all the intricate movements humans make. In a later chapter, I will explain these relationships and manipulation.

It is for this reason, that chiropractors adjust more regions than just your lumbar spine, to restore normal function to your lower back. Often, if your ankles are pronated or supinated, Orthotics that fit in your shoes will be fitted.

Chiropractors are usually quite holistic in their philosophy and will be concerned about your diet and lifestyle. Fast foods don't supply the micro and macro nutrients that the body needs to heal properly.

To ensure that the chiropractor you choose is up-to-date and practicing modern concepts, a list of questions follows. The information enclosed in brackets gives the underlying reasons for asking the questions.

1. Will you conduct tests to rule out a systemic cause of my back pain, if your consultation and examination indicates it is necessary?
2. Will you take x-rays no bigger than 14 inches by 17 inches or will you send me out to a radiologist. Don't allow a full spine 14 x 36 inches picture to be taken unless a scoliosis is suspected. If the films are taken in house, ask for them to be sent out for reading by a chiropractic or medical radiologist for a written report. (It will cost more, but it is worth it. This will assure that the film quality is good and that a bone pathology is not overlooked.)
3. Will you be trying to correct misalignments? Or will you be restoring mechanical function to my joints? (Manipulation has little effect on realigning the spine. Manipulation does restore range of motion and joint function.)
4. Do you treat and restore function to my sacroiliacs, hips, knees and ankles for lower back pain if needed? (Do not accept treatment only to your lower back. The cause of

your low back inflammation and pain is often lower in the locomotor chain of joints and muscles.)

5. What is your diagnosis? Write it down. (At this point remember the four types of mechanical causes. Don't accept the cause as a "misaligned bone pinching a nerve. A pinched, compressed nerve radiates pain down from your back and causes tingling or numbness and weakness. Check the diagnosis you are given against the test questions in Chapter 2. If you have numbness and weakness etc. you should be sent for special tests to make sure surgery is not necessary. Some patients without insurance coverage can't afford an MRI and we do a 6 to 8 weeks clinical trial to see if a favorable response occurs. If not a surgical consultation is arranged.
6. After my pain subsides, will you provide or arrange for rehabilitation of the soft tissue flexibility and strengthening to prevent further attacks. (Prevention is not getting adjusted every month without doing your exercises and stretches, unless the degenerative changes are too advanced)
7. If I have degenerative discs and chronic changes, will I be provided with regular monthly care to assure that joint locking and muscle spasms are kept to a minimum. (Prevention and spinal management are important chiropractic services often misunderstood by well meaning critics of chiropractic. For some chronic sufferers it improves their quality of life dramatically to be compared to daily insulin for diabetics. Neither is a cure but great management strategies.)
8. What is the therapy for the inflammation, and what part of the treatment is working toward restoring spinal function? (Manipulation should be given where the joints are

locked (blocked), very often not at the point where your back hurts. Physical therapy, such as interferential electro therapy, applied at the painful, inflamed areas speeds up the recovery. Manipulation of the inflamed area can keep it sore and inflamed. It is very common to need different adjustments or manipulation in different areas of the spine and extremities to get your spine back to normal.)

I am a chiropractor who has made the paradigm shift. This description of what a chiropractor does, is not describing some of the off-shoots of mainline Chiropractic. My goal is to make you an informed consumer, who knows something of their problem. Knowing this, gives you the ability to recognize, if the brand of chiropractic being offered to you, makes sense.

This book will be boycotted by many chiropractors, because they want you to believe you have a misaligned spine. Beware of some, who ask for thousands of dollars up front, to cover a years' care, needed to realign your spine. Their adjustments will increase the function of your joints, just like all other manipulations. Their good results are not from realigning your spine, even if they say it is so. Two x-ray studies done in Europe showed only 12% of spines look better on x-rays after treatment. If you are shown some examples, they were purposely selected and not randomly chosen from all, past cases. Be an informed consumer; go to one of the thousands of skilled chiropractors out there, who understand the functional paradigm.

Massage Therapists

Licensed massage therapists normally work in cooperation with other practitioners as part of an overall back pain management program. Massage is especially helpful in the treatment of muscle spasms, congested muscles, blocked lymphatic drainage, and fascia constrictions and adhesions.

Massage offers both physiological and psychological benefits. Therapists can ease or prevent muscle spasms, stimulate blood and lymphatic circulation, and offer soothing, calming effects by stroking the surface of the body. A therapeutic massage is often effective in speeding up the recovery, by reversing established muscle contractions that won't let go. Rolfing and near Rolfing massage methods are deep tissue, techniques, that stretch the muscle fibers and the fascia surrounding the muscles. It hurts, but it is very helpful.

There are sub-groups within this category of massage therapists, and almost as many techniques as technicians. Basic to all techniques, is that the muscle is massaged sideways to separate the fibers and fascia, or stripped length-wise to elongate the muscle cells and stretch any shortening adhesions. Another purpose is to milk toxic by-products from injury or even excessive exercise.

If you are considering going to a massage therapist, or if your doctor recommends massage, make sure you know the purpose of the massage and the type of massage you are going to get. Is it prescribed to help you relax and feel good or is it therapeutic to break up adhesions, free up adhesions between nerves and their coverings, reduce congestion or create lymphatic drainage? They are all different and everyone needs to be on the same page.

The doctor might be expecting one outcome and the massage therapist another. Make sure you know what you are getting massage for and that you receive the right kind.

Osteopaths

There are two different schools of osteopathy. The first is the more traditional approach, wherein the osteopath is a specialist in manipulation, and can determine the different causes of back pain. The second type is the modern osteopath. Usually, this person is the equivalent of a medical doctor who has received limited training in manipulation techniques. They can offer treatments combining drugs, surgery and a limited version of the traditional, osteopathic manipulations.

Mechanical back pain patients should seek the osteopathic practitioner using conservative methods, but do not duplicate the services of a medical doctor. Some osteopaths use muscle energy and cranial pressure techniques that are more esoteric. Once again make sure your mechanical problems are receiving attention. There is no magic system. It is always all about removing all the mechanical causes. Here is a list of pertinent questions you should ask an osteopath:

1. Are you primarily practicing osteopathic manipulation, with drugs and surgery as a back-up?
2. Will or have you had sufficient tests to rule out systemic causes of back pain?
3. If x-rays were taken, have they been read by a specialist in reading x-rays? Remember paying a little more is much better than having them taken and read in any doctors' office.
4. What is my diagnosis?
5. How will the inflammation be treated and how will the dysfunctional problems be treated?

6. Once the pain goes away, what care will follow at home or in a gym?
7. If you don't do manipulation on a regular basis, can you recommend a practitioner who can restore normal function to the locked joints?

Acupuncturists

These practitioners work on the theory that a back pain is caused by an imbalance in the bodies' meridian system. Meridian lines have been charted on the body by ancient Chinese practitioners to illustrate acupuncture points. Each meridian represents an organ such as the Liver Meridian. The theory is that the Chi energy gets blocked and the placement of needles restores the flow and balance of energy along the meridians. In the western world of science, energy does not flow and the meridians can not be measured. In spite of the ancient explanation, this treatment can often be effective in relieving pain. Western research has found that when these needles are inserted, endorphins are released. Endorphins are hormones produced by the brain which have a potent pain-killing effect.

As the pain is relieved, the back sufferer can attain a much better range of motion, which in turn can break the vicious spasm-pain-muscle spasm cycle. This occurs not because the meridians have been balanced, but because the pain has been arrested via the production of endorphins.

The above is a very simplistic explanation of how the acupuncturist can help treat bad backs. Sufferers must be aware that there are many causes of back pain, and they must recognize that many causes would not respond to acupuncture in the long run.

Unfortunately, the field of acupuncture is cluttered with poorly-trained, inexperienced, over-zealous practitioners. Neither a few weekends nor a few hundred hours is long enough for a person to become a specialist. If you seek an acupuncturist make sure that they are adequately qualified and display the letters L. Ac.Dipl. Ac. These acupuncturists have had a four year post-graduate course of study.

Remember, too, that for long lasting relief, the poor mechanics you have been reading about must be corrected. If the acupuncturist does not lengthen your hamstring muscles or send you to get your sacroiliac joint freed up, for example, you are destined for another back pain episode. The second question is, will your chosen acupuncturist do the necessary examination procedures to discover a systemic condition. Masking over the pain, may allow a bone disease to go undiscovered. In my opinion, east must meet west, when it comes to the diagnosis and treatment of back pain.

Podiatrists

If your back pain originates in the legs or feet, then this specialist may be able to successfully treat the condition by placing an orthotic device inside your shoe. Specially, if you have "sloping in" of the ankle, which is called Pronation and is a mechanical cause of back pain, a podiatrist can help. The orthotic the podiatrist makes to order, can take the torque off your knee and low back.

Pronation causes the knee and upper leg to rotate forward and inward as well. This forward rotation also carries the pelvis forward on the same side. Walking around with this problem produces a mechanical insult every time the opposite swinging leg tries to rotate the pelvis forward. An average person takes 20,000 to 30,000 of these steps every day. This mechanical stress wears away on your lower back, like the Colorado River gouging out the Grand Canyon. Only, it doesn't take a million years to happen in our spine.

Informed back pain sufferers should be able to determine if they are candidates for Orthotics through their own self-examinations. Otherwise, it would be ridiculous, costly and perhaps even detrimental for a patient to wear Orthotics if there were no existing condition to justify it.

Remember, to determine whether there is Pronation or Supination look at your ankles from behind. You will need a mirror or a friend to look from behind. Each Achilles tendon should be perpendicular to the floor. The tendon's ridge at the back of your ankle should be straight up from the floor; not angling inwards or outwards.

Temporary Orthotics or taping of the affected area, can often determine whether a patient will respond to this type of treatment, thereby avoiding the unnecessary costs of a useless, permanent appliance, which can run as high as $1,200.00. You should never pay more than $400.00. Ask your back specialist to confirm if you have ankle deviation from the perpendicular.

In the past few years, there has been a movement away from posting the heel with the appliance and going to an appliance that torques the long axis of the foot to achieve a correction. The reason this newer method is preferred, is that the foot and ankle in mid stance, during walking, the ankle needs to pronate a little. The old Orthotics, that used a wedge at the heel, prevented any Pronation during walking and running. Again it is a matter of preserving function and not just correcting the Pronation while standing still. The paradigm has also shifted in this field, just like in Chiropractic.

Allergists

Sometimes back pain is caused by an adverse reaction to a particular food, beverage or airborne, toxic chemical. It is not completely understood how allergies can manifest themselves as back pain, joint pain or the stiffening of the musculature, but they do. The allergen is a stressor to your system and triggers the release of chemicals that increases any inflammation anywhere in the body. A low grade, low back strain becomes a full fledged inflamed, posterior, back joint inflammation. The pain, muscle spasm, more pain cycle commences all from a hidden allergy. Fortunately, there are ways to determine whether an allergy is the cause or not.

One way is a four-day fast, undertaken, of course, with the doctor's supervision. During this fast, the patient drinks only water and a bit of fruit juice (hopefully a fruit you are not allergic to). The water fast removes all the food allergies from the system; quite often by the fourth day, all the aches and pains are also gone! In this way you can determine whether or not you are suffering from back pain caused by an allergic reaction to food. Unfortunately, a water fast will not help the majority of back pain sufferers.

If the pain is caused by an allergy, then the allergist will know what to do. In these cases, experience has shown me that coffee is a common culprit for people suffering with muscle spasms and pain between their shoulder blades.

Don't do this fast unsupervised. Sometimes salt and sugar needs to be supplemented to avoid a health crisis. That is why a little juice is recommended instead of just water. If the 4 day fast clears up your back pain, make an appointment with an allergist or holistic health practitioner who orders allergy tests to determine exactly what are your allergies.

Nutritionists

In the past year research is coming out that has shown some foods are very pro-inflammatory and not in an allergic way. Modern science can now look at the remains of our forefathers from 10,000 years ago and analyze what they used to eat. The long and short of the story is that they did not eat any grains. Following on from that, grains have an abundance of Omega 6 oils and not enough Omega 3 oils. Omega 6 oils feed the inflammation cascade. Omega 3 oils are anti-inflammatory. We always knew that halibut and cod liver oil helped reduce the pain of arthritic joints, especially if Vitamin C was present in sufficient quantities.

Vitamin C is a very unstable substance and it is destroyed by heat and oxidation. Squeeze it yourself, fresh every day from citrus fruit. Supermarket, orange juice is days old and has been oxidized in the big juicers they use to press out the juice. It loses a lot of the vitamin C in the process. Vitamin C is used by the body to maintain our connective tissue and heal inflammation. If you are a slow healer, you may need more Vitamin C in your diet. Smoking one cigarette destroys the amount of vitamin C in one ripe orange. It is not easy to eat one orange for every cigarette, if you smoke.

The electrolyte minerals can also be deficient and cause muscle spasms, weakness and ultimately back pain and cramping of the muscles. Many chiropractors give their patients nutritional supplements to make sure no deficiencies are occurring. Some patients prefer to see a nutritionist and make life-style changes to their diet.

It is not commonly understood, that some deficiencies take months of supplementation before the body's cells are no longer deficient. For example, one experiment with long term prisoners, given a zinc deficient diet until they were zinc deficient, discovered it took six months on zinc supplements to get back to normal, cellular, zinc counts. It can be in the blood quite quickly, but take a while to get inside your cells.

Assays of fresh foods today have 35 to 50% less vitamins and minerals compared to foods assayed just after the Second World War. In those days crops were grown in manure fertilized fields, where the soil was alive with bacterial activity. Today western farmers can chemically fertilize sandy soil and grow two or three crops a year. It is not the same and we have the taste buds to prove it. Many of the modern fruits and vegetables are tasteless by comparison. Whole Food Markets and some Farmers Markets do their best to provide nutritious old fashioned produce. Organic labels mean no systemic pesticides have been used in the growing process. You can't wash off these chemicals; they are designed to go inside the fruits and vegetables to ward off attacks and prolong shelf-life.

If your response to treatment for your back is puzzling your provider; consider looking at the nutritional factor.

Psychiatrists/Psychologists

When anxiety amplifies the magnitude of the pain, or when there is any other type of psychological component to the sufferer's back problem, then the patient should be receiving counseling from a psychiatrist or psychologist. This counseling is most effective when done in conjunction with treatment from a back specialist.

When the stress is self-inflicted you can correct the situation yourself. If the cause of your stress and anxiety are not apparent, then you need professional help. Ask your prime practitioner to refer you to a capable psychotherapist, who is interested in holistic health care.

It has been known for many years that people that are unhappy with their jobs suffer from back pain and are much more difficult to help than those who are happy at work. It has been shown that patients with a high degree of job satisfaction overcome their back injuries and surgeries better and faster than those who are unhappy with their vocations. Back pain can cause reactive depression which almost always disappears when the pain goes away. However chronic depression or anxiety can impede or make a full recovery unobtainable.

A good clinical psychologist can do a psychological survey and let you know if counseling is needed for a permanent recovery, void of episodes.

Don't be embarrassed, as this type of complication can be the start of the stresses destroying your general health.

Yoga

Most back exercises prescribed by specialists are derived from yoga. Body movement involves muscle strength, muscle and other soft tissue flexibility, physical endurance and balance. Exercise machines increase muscle strength and endurance. Stretching exercises elongate muscles and increase the elasticity of tendons, ligaments and other connective soft tissues. But yoga does it all, improving strength, endurance, flexibility and balance. The reason this form of exercise is performed with bare feet standing, lying and upside down is to impose a demand on the automatically controlled (not consciously controlled) postural muscles. Yoga also offers a serenity and philosophy that controls stress and promotes a natural, healthful lifestyle.

Many yoga postures create leverages which can cause spontaneous joint manipulation. I find it is best to release the blockages with a skilled manipulator and then go on to yoga. The problem with spontaneous manipulations is that they often cause an adjustment at the inflamed and already mobile joint. They "pop" because the joint gaps not because a correction has necessarily been achieved.

This is why so many experienced yoga masters work with a competent chiropractor who performs the specific manipulation needed. The motion palpation many doctors learn is ideal for detecting the spinal and extremity joint blockages. It should also be stated that once a chiropractor achieves a mobile, pain free spine; he or she should recommend that the patient should work to achieve strong, flexible muscles and ligaments as well as to activate the balancing responses.

Yoga is a wonderful method of achieving these desired results. Don't be aggressive, go gently and take your time. It is best to avoid end range static positions. End range loading is the most common cause of sprains and strains. You can't speed up nature's response to an imposed demand. An over zealous stretch will cause an injury. Don't let anyone physically place there hands on you and push you further into a posture. I have seen a lot of injuries as a result of a yoga instructor pushing and spraining a clients' back. Yoga results take months and years to achieve, unless you are less than 25 years old.

Back Schools

Back schools of about four or five lectures and workshops have been shown to help considerably, in removing the stress and anxiety of back pain sufferers. The schools also teach good posture, lifting skills, exercises and basic movements of sitting, lifting, walking and sleeping.

Back classes usually are recommended after a successful treatment plan by many different practitioners. Patients who attend these schools receive the necessary information applicable to changing bad habits and lifestyles that have been major causes of their back pain.

These classes are usually run by a physiotherapist in hospitals, community centers, YMCA or church halls. The cost is low because they can have eight or ten to a class. The success rate is so good that many insurance companies will cover the cost. Some employers teach their at-risk employees how to protect their backs on the job.

Hopefully, reading this book will serve as a kind of back school program for you.

Chapter Four

The Therapies

"If it seems ridiculous ....it probably is."

There are many accepted therapeutic methods to stop back pain. Some are temporary pain relievers. Some remove the causal factors. Still others keep the patient occupied and satisfied as the body heals in spite of the intervention. In previous chapters, you have been able to identify your condition or conditions and now you can see what treatment will suit you best.

Drug Therapy

On the surface, this therapy would appear to be the easiest way to get relief from back problems. Unfortunately, drugs can't change the causal factors. As well as kill the pain they carry the risk of side effects which are oftentimes much worse and more debilitating than the original back pain.

Drug therapy is divided into three main groups: 1. The Anti-inflammatories, 2. The Pain Relievers, 3. The Muscle Relaxants. Sometimes an anti-depressant is prescribed.

The Anti-inflammatory Drugs

The anti-inflammatory drugs are steroids (such as cortisone) or non-steroidal (such as ibuprofen, the ingredient in Motrin and Advil).

The steroids have the most serious side effects and should not be accepted as treatment unless there is severe, incapacitating pain or previous, therapeutic failures. Their side effects can cause serious demineralization of the bones and fluid retention which leads to other health problems.

The non-steroidal drugs, such as Motrin and aspirin, are very effective at reducing inflammation. Yet, some studies show that their use over an extended period of time can also alter the healing process. Tissues that heal with anti-inflammatories look different than tissues that heal naturally. Under a microscope the cells are disorganized and not polarized like they should be. This leads to easier re-injury and the prolonged need for more anti-inflammatories. They do not deal with the cause of the inflammation and if taken for years, they accelerate the degeneration. It is like not re-aligning the wheels on your car and just dealing with the tires.

The Pain Killers

Pain killers such as aspirin and acetaminophen should only be used on a short term basis. The theory behind taking pain killers is to deaden the pain enough to allow better joint movement, and hence increase joint function. This, in turn, will stimulate nerve endings, blocking the pain response, and also relax the spastic muscles. The body can then get on with healing itself, especially if the cause of the pain is corrected.

The Muscle Relaxants

Muscle relaxants have been a disappointment. Research studies have shown they do not help a low back pain patient to any significant amount.

They are often prescribed with the pain killers and anti-inflammatories. In theory they should help reduce the muscle spasm and in turn reduce the pain caused by the muscle spasm. There is some evidence that drug therapy combined with manipulation is better than either one on its own. It is my experience that many of my patients take something, either over the counter or prescription strength.

General practitioners and chiropractors working together can achieve marvelous results. As the patient you must orchestrate this approach yourself. More family practitioners are now familiar with modern, rational spinal and extremity joint manipulation. By the same token, modern chiropractors are not against the use of short-term drug therapy to reduce pain and inflammation. If you have two reasonable and rational doctors to whom you suggest cooperative therapy management, you will get pain relief and the mechanical problem solved. They may even learn to treat other patients the same way if they are not already doing so.

Never be afraid to take matters of health into your own hands. Doctors take an oath to help the patient foremost. Beware of the doctor who has an ego too big to allow cooperative effort. He's probably just out for monetary gain, at yours and other patients' expense.

Cold Packs

These are the simplest home remedy for anti-inflammation reduction, muscle relaxation and pain relief. But be forewarned, you should not apply ice on the painful area for more than 15 minutes at a time. Otherwise, the tissue will become too chilled and the body will send more blood to warm up the tissue. Over chilling like heat encourages swelling by increasing the size of the small blood vessels called capillaries. In essence, it reverses reduction of the swelling and inflammation that the initial cold pack produces. It's better to apply the ice for 10 to 12 minutes, remove it for an hour, and then apply it again for another 12 minutes. You will find this gives you the best and safest home remedy for anti-inflammatory care.

You may have wondered why the gel packs you chill for applying a cold pack is so thin. These have been designed to chill for the twelve minutes and not longer like ice cubes. It is also good to know, that if you put these gel packs in the refrigerator and not the freezer, you can place them on the bare skin without any protective insulation. They are just as effective and you won't get a freezer burn.

If you use crushed ice or ice cubes, put water in the bag with the ice. This will conform to irregular surfaces and will not burn either. Remember 12 minutes only, every hour.

Manipulation

History of the Technique

It appears that man knew almost instinctively that manipulation helped ease back pain. Manipulation of the spine and extremity joints dates back before recorded time. Mayan pottery sculptures depict individuals being stretched and pushed upon. Cave dweller's wall art clearly shows people being manipulated, as do the earliest writing tablets. It was crude then, but obviously it helped.

Around the Sixth Century A.D., manipulation fell into ill repute. A powerful Roman pope of the time decreed that surgery and manipulation were heresy. Punishable by death, no less! Surgery was the first of these two techniques to come out of the dark ages, while manipulation got its emancipation in the late eighteen hundreds.

A self-educated Canadian by the name of Daniel Palmer developed chiropractic. Simultaneously, around 1885, a medical doctor named Andrew Still developed osteopathy. Both osteopathy and chiropractic became full-fledged professions, in spite of heavy opposition from the medical community, which included the use of some illegal tactics by medical doctors who felt threatened by the new sciences. In the famous 1989 Wilkes case in Illinois, the American Medical Association (AMA) was found guilty of using illegal tactics against chiropractic. To oppose osteopathic medicine, they absorbed them and then diminished the importance of manipulation in osteopathic care.

Recently, in most countries of the world, these old battles have been completely forgotten. The education level of chiropractors has raised so significantly, that their research is now being widely published. Some papers have even appeared in the prestigious Spine Journal. Here in the U.S., many inter-disciplinary societies and conferences continue to develop, and the necessary exchange of important scientific information is occurring. Within the American Back Society, orthopedists, chiropractors, physiotherapists, and osteopaths meet twice a year for three days of lectures and workshops.

Rational dialogue and cooperation are leading to better treatment for patients suffering from a multitude of nerve, muscle and bone disorders. Athletes and weekend warriors alike are also finding they can overcome injuries and achieve better performance with the help of manipulation.

I was appointed by the Canadian Government to be with the Olympic Track and Field Team for the 1984 Olympics, held in Los Angeles. Coordination of movement for the elite performance of a sport is best when all the nerve endings in the joints are able to report back to the brain that the movements needed, are occurring. Muscles are recruited smoothly and efficiently, if no compensations are employed. Slightly dysfunctional feet, ankles, knees or hips can change an elite runners' performance. Our pentathlon entry was going to be unable to participate if I had not restored function to the superior tibular-fibula joint, at the side of his knee. The knee pain cleared in 3 days and he had time to continue training at the pre-Olympic training camp in Sacramento. As you know Olympic athletes have to be drug free to compete fairly. He needed to be pain free and able to bend his knee, in order to be able to compete at all.

How the Technique Works

The joint space is enclosed by a capsular sac containing the joint fluid. This fluid lubricates the slippery surfaces and supplies nutrients in a blood free zone. Manipulation or "adjustment" as chiropractors term it, is the physical separation of the joint space. When the joint surfaces are separated by just a few millimeters, the area (volume) of the joint space is increased, thus lowering the pressure on the fluids inside the joint.

When your chiropractor performs manipulation, a cracking sound is often heard as gases pop out of the joint fluids. This is the same phenomenon as gas bubbles appearing in a bottle of soda when the cap is removed. Once this cavitation has occurred, the joint can glide on this nitrogen and carbon dioxide gas bubble for 20 minutes before it is reabsorbed. The nerves that record movement are reactivated and the messages sent to your brain are used to recruit muscles that move the same joint. This new activity of restored motion in the joint starts a series of recuperative events.

The most rational approach to manipulation is to adjust the joint with the lost range of motion, not the inflamed joint producing the pain. Years ago at an interdisciplinary conference where I presented a lecture on the topic, the panel of experts came to the consensus that manipulation should be used as part of the strategy to remove the cause of mechanical dysfunction. Doctors from varied professions confirmed that one should not manipulate inflamed joints. The skilled chiropractor or osteopath should manipulate the locked joints anywhere in the locomotor system, above, below and opposite the inflamed back joint. Sometimes the major restriction is in a hip, knee or ankle joint.

Manipulation should be repeated daily or every other day at first, until all ranges of motion are restored. Full recovery of the lost ranges of motion is usually achieved after the pain has stopped in the nearby inflamed area of the spine. As the inflamed joint improves and it also starts to move better the nerve endings called mechanoreceptors are activated. If the brain is receiving these messages it will ignore the pain messages from the pain, nociceptor, nerve endings and your pain will be much less. It is for this reason manipulation can reduce pain as well as start the return back to a full range of motion between the vertebrae.

Manipulation removes a major cause of back pain, which is the blockage or lack of normal function in a joint that can not be restored by exercising or stretching. It is a shame so many sufferers are exercising with abnormal function and thus establishing pain-free compensations. These compensations will lead to more serious degenerative complications, as we saw with the aerobics instructor in Chapter One. "Manipulation first and exercise later" is what I always recommend. Used in this sequence, the exercise helps maintain the normal biomechanics needed for a pain-free, episode-free lower back.

Manipulation must not be a war between the forces of the manipulator and the holding elements of a joint. The best manipulation is a pleasant experience as the sense of tension is released.

Occasionally a healing crisis occurs after a manipulation. This is like a fever which peaks right before it breaks – you perspire profusely, and then feel much better. Although this crisis can be painful, most of the pain and inflammation disappears after 24 to 48 hours. Good reactions to a manipulation are a general flood of mild perspiration over your entire body, and a feeling of warmth. Sometimes you need to take a big breath in and just let yourself go. Patients often get very sleepy after the first few treatments; it is best to give in and go home and have a healing nap. Almost everyone has a great sense of well being, because the spine feels good when it is loose and mobile.

Experience has shown me that everyone could benefit from having at least two full spine and extremity manipulations every year. The caveat to this is that you need to make sure your doctor is only manipulating the joints he or she finds locked or blocked. This can prevent faulty biomechanical compensations from developing. Cracking normal joints is not preventing anything. Even though there is no evidence that manipulation harms normal joints, only the locked joints should be adjusted. Unlocking the dysfunctional joints in the directions they are restricted affects the coordination of the whole locomotor system. Adjusting an already mobile joint is like cracking your knuckles, nothing changes. Manipulation increases motion in hypo mobile joints: motion promotes proper healing.

Electrotherapy

There are many different varieties of electrotherapy, some more effective than others for treating back pain. Electrotherapy utilizes machines which produce a very mild electric current from an electrode pad placed on the surface of the skin. Some currents kill pain, and some reduce swelling and inflammation, while others strengthen weakened muscles. In my experience, the most comfortable and effective for doing all of the above is an interferential machine.

Interferential electrotherapy is applied by placing four carbon, self-sticking pads all around the area of inflammation in your back. Two mild cross-currents somewhat out of phase with each other create a three dimensional electric field that encompasses the inflamed tissues. This electric field can be controlled by varying the difference between the two currents. The most effective anti-inflammatory, pain-relieving effects are achieved by currents that prickle the skin as they pass through, but are not strong enough to cause any muscle contractions. Each application lasts from 10 to 15 minutes. Any less will not give the patient the optimum benefit of the treatment, and any more is superfluous.

These mild currents have multiple beneficial effects and replace the need for other electrotherapy that achieves only one specific reaction. With interferential the circulation is increased, the swelling reduced, the pain deadened, the healing process speeded up, and the weakened muscles are strengthened. Nothing replaces the overall multiple effects of interferential electrotherapy when properly applied. It can be applied more than once daily to reduce inflammation and swelling. To strengthen atrophied or deconditioned muscles it takes 24 hours to fully respond to one application.

The little cell phone, sized units you may see advertised are not the same as the professional, much bigger units that are used in doctors and physiotherapists' offices.

TENS is another form of electrotherapy. It is a small, portable unit and is specifically designed to reduce pain. You may have tried one or seen someone wearing a small power pack on their belt. It looks like a pager with wires attached. The stick-on electrodes at the end of the wire are placed near the spine, where the prickling of the skin by the pulsing or constant current is emitted to block the pain. The sensation and stimulation of the sensory nerves overrides the nociceptors, (pain nerve endings) and replaces the pain sensation with a prickly skin sensation. For some patients this is welcomed relief until other treatment is effective.

Beware of the ridiculous cost some sellers are asking for these little, portable units. Comparison shop on the internet. They range from $39.00 to $200.00 and they are basically all the same if they have passed our government safety approval. Don't buy one that does not have the safety stamp.

Ultrasound

The ultrasound machine uses a very high frequency, radio crystal to transmit sound waves through your skin into the painful area of your back or muscles. The most up to date ultrasound machines have solved all the side effect problems of units made years ago. Areas of congested hyaluronic acid called "Trigger Points" are easily treated with the application of ultrasound over the trigger point area of the muscle. Muscle trigger points are quite common and spray and stretch used to be the method of choice for treatment. The methane spray is very bad for the atmosphere and its' use is much less common now.

Balancing Exercises

Although gymnastics, yoga and other traditional exercise systems challenge the balance mechanisms, back pain sufferers in general do not participate in such activities to achieve their benefits. Research from former Communist Eastern bloc countries researched the effectiveness of spending a few minutes each day on rocker and balancing boards. These studies reveal that balancing exercises cause marked changes in the function of the important automatically controlled deep, smaller, back muscles.

In the past 20 years these methods have gravitated to the West. Back pain specialists and body movement instructors have devised unique and fun filled ways to develop our balance reflexes and strengthen our Core muscles.

Yoga is always practiced in bare feet, which stimulates all the nerve endings normally harnessed in hard-soled shoes. Even running shoes are a restriction to all the foot movement that can occur in your bare feet.

The use of a large exercise ball for "Ball Exercises" is another popular method of doing a workout with an unstable base. All the book stores sell soft backed books on how to do the ball exercises, all of which can be done at home.

The balls come in 55cm, 65cm, 75cm sizes and a hand or foot pump to inflate them to almost hard; leave a little give in them. Don't be frugal, the cheap ones burst when you bounce on them. If you buy one that has to be inflated at the gas station, you may get a surprise after it is filled. It could be too big to get into the trunk or back seat of your car. I have had a few laughs with patients in the past, when they met this dilemma.

Pilates exercise routines are performed on a machine and is less likely to challenge your balance, unless the Pilates instructor works with you off the "Rack" as it is fondly nicknamed.

The weight training machines isolate muscles, so that you can control the muscles you wish to workout, each session. These machines do not challenge the balance mechanisms. Obviously you must add balance exercises to a machine, dominant workout.

The rule is to get rid of the inflammation and pain, before you start any exercise program. You should learn a stretch routine as well, before you exercise. If you have been inactive with your back pain for more than three months, your back muscles will be deconditioned. They may even be filled with fat, which is called fatty degeneration. Reconditioning will reverse these changes but be patient, never strain to lift more like a body builder. Body builders have healthy, strong muscles not deconditioned.

Surgery

If you are reading this book because you are being advised to have surgery, you have many more choices than a surgical candidate of even five years ago. Today the surgeons make much smaller incisions and the recovery times are much shorter. These smaller incisions don't do the extensive damage to surrounding tissues, like the larger ones.

Surgeons are not suggesting laminectomies and fusions of the vertebrae and back joints like before. These surgeries had a high rate of poor outcomes and often a second and even a third surgery was needed in a segment above. Today they can go in and pare the disc or trim a bony spur or even place a separator, to relieve compressive stenosis. Now discs can be replaced with ball bearing-like discs. These disc replacement apparatuses preserve the motion between the two vertebrae and are predicted to avoid the need for second surgeries, previously needed after fusions.

It is estimated about three percent of chronic back pain patients need surgery. Most surgeons today recommend conservative care first. The problem is they often have an irrational bias to manipulation. This bias often prevents a patient from success, with conservative chiropractic care. Happily, I can say, more and more surgeons are getting familiar with rational, skillful, manipulators in their community.

Let the Buyer Beware

There is no need for you to become a classic, back pain sufferer. If your doctor becomes upset with you, for being an informed consumer of his health care, then go elsewhere. It will, more than likely, take a team to get you pain free and rehabilitated. You will not alter this disease process by a single action of any one of the following:

- Taking pain killers.
- Sticking needles in your back or along the liver median.
- Getting back manipulation or mobilization.
- Getting your back tapped by a spring loaded hammer.
- Meditating daily.
- Hanging upside down daily.
- Wearing an orthopedic support belt.
- Having an orthotic device placed in your shoe.
- Avoid lifting, bending or twisting.
- Applying heat packs and ultrasound
- Wearing a red flannel band around your waste.

- Lying on wedge shaped blocks or dense foam rolls.
- Working out at a gym with weight machines
- Getting the knots massaged
- Etc., etc., etc.

At best, these treatments provide temporary relief unless you change the accumulated, mechanical dysfunction, after getting pain relief.

Chapter Five

Home Treatment

"One-third knowledge and inspiration, one-third perspiration, and one-third worry-free relaxation"

The most important rule for successful treatment of back pain is to obtain the correct diagnosis. This rule holds true for home as well as professional care. Make sure you understand the previous chapters on self-diagnosis, the specialists and the therapies before you begin treating yourself at home. Since 10% of back pain is not mechanical in origin, delaying the correct diagnosis could prove fatal. Bone cancers need to be diagnosed earlier rather than later.

Therapeutic Goals of Home Treatment

You will be aiming for several therapeutic goals by home treatment of your back pain. These include:

- Reducing pain.
- Reducing inflammation.
- Reducing swelling.
- Promoting healing of primary tissue.
- Discouraging adhesive scar tissue formation.

- Increasing the passive and active ranges of back motion by stretching.
- Increasing back strength.
- Increasing the strength of supportive abdominal and pelvic muscles referred to as the Core Muscles.
- Increasing the passive ranges of motion of the ligaments.
- Improving posture.
- Improving lifting methods.
- Reducing stress factors.
- Reducing the body fat-to-muscle ratio.
- Learning an effective relaxation technique.
- Stop fearing and worrying about back pain once you know it is mechanical and not a systemic disease. The fear and worry creates muscle spasm and chronicity.

You should already be sharing many of these goals with your doctor or therapist, and achieving greater results with their help. However, if you can also be carrying out rational, intelligent home care; you can help yourself speed up the healing process. It is interesting to note that studies show that bed rest is the worst thing you can do, as it prolongs your recovery. Let's examine each of these goals individually.

Reducing Pain

If you feel you have sprained or strained your back, the best remedy is ice or a cold pack. Never use heat. Don't even take a hot shower. Heat has been shown to delay the recovery of any sprain by three weeks. Take a quick, lukewarm shower instead of your usual hot shower.

For best results apply an ice pack or cold gel pack for 10 to 12 minutes every hour, especially the first several hours after the injury. Place the ice directly over the most painful area. This will restrict the swelling, lessen the pain, reduce the reactive muscle spasm and speed up the overall recovery process. Using ice or a cold pack quickly and repeatedly as described above is time well spent. Don't ever avoid this step. Do not leave the ice on more than 12 minutes at a time. It is the repeated act of cooling, after it warms up for an hour that is the therapeutic part. Leaving ice on for much longer has the opposite effect and only gives you one cooling action instead of repeated cooling effects.

You may have heard that you only need to ice for the first 24 hours. This is erroneous, you need to ice as long s it is inflamed and swollen.

The old remedy of bed rest for strain or sprain has proven to be the worst thing you can do. It actually delays recovery. When you have pain, it is advisable to refrain from normal activity. But be sure to keep varying your postures from lying on one side, to sitting, standing, kneeling, walking, lying on your back with the calves of your legs over a chair to lying face down, etc. Lying face down with your elbows on the floor and your hands propping up your head and neck is often a relieving position. (See Figure 6.)

Most over-the-counter pain killers help reduce pain, but they have been proven to interfere with the healing process with extended use. Some topical creams, salves and ointments create a cold sensation on the skin to distract you away from pain. Others contain aspirin or capsicum, which are anti-inflammatories as well as pain killers.

To a small degree, pain can be controlled by a TENS unit which is variable, electrical output. The body can very quickly become accustomed to a constant, electrical, output level and then the pain killing effect is lost. If I sound somewhat skeptical it's because I have never seen very good results from the use of a TENS unit.

Reducing Inflammation and Swelling

Inflammation is the body's response to injury. It is designed to ward off and restrict bacterial infections from gaining access to the bloodstream. This is great, except that in 99.9% of back pain injuries there is no infection to wall off. So the sooner the inflammatory process can be stopped and dissipated, the better.

There are a myriad of prescription and over-the-counter anti-inflammatory drugs which effectively reduce inflammation. However, the real secret to reducing inflammation is to use an ice or gel pack, which has no side effects. Swelling should be reduced as soon as possible with ice or a cold gel pack. Yet, for most back pain sufferers the swelling is not apparent, because it is internal. The main exception is the sacroiliac joints which often swell quite visibly. Use ice packs as explained above as often as possible. Repeating the cooling process is best.

Promoting Healing of the Primary Tissue

To promote the healing of the primary tissue, you must supply your body with the micro and macro nutrients it needs. It is vital to increase your intake of vitamin C, and to eat plenty of fresh fruits and vegetables (preferably raw or only blanched). If it is difficult for you to spend a few minutes in the sunshine every day, be sure to supplement your diet with a natural fish oil containing Vitamin D.

The foods rich in Omega 3 oils act as an anti-inflammatory and help healing naturally. Too many grains will increase your Omega 6 intake and have the effect of increasing your pro-inflammatory hormones, which delay tissues from healing.

Rest promotes healing; don't exercise your back if it causes pain lasting a few seconds. Stop the moment you feel any pain and resume the exercise another day.

This is no time to be macho, stop even half way through an exercise, don't force yourself to finish. If you try to work/exercise through pain then you are re-enforcing bad/compensatory movement patterns and increasing compensatory muscle patterning.

Rest promotes healing but staying in bed for a few days has been shown to delay your recovery. Rest means relax, keep changing your postures. Kneel, sit, stand, stretch, lie face up, face down or on your side. Move every twenty 20 minutes, the pain free postures should be favored.

Ice is always better than heat even though heat is comforting.

Discouraging Adhesive Scar Tissue Formation

When the pain is no longer acute and you are in the healing process, it is important to isolate movement and stretches in the previous painful area. Don't let the healing occur with a shortened muscle condition.

Your body will repair the tissue by following natural laws. Tissue will be supplied to fulfill the need of the imposed demand. If the demand is movement, then normal and elastic tissue will regenerate. If you only rest, the demand for immobility is the imposed demand, adhesions will develop and a second-rate healing job will result.

These different types of healing responses have been shown by researchers more than twenty years ago. The result of their findings led to motorized, joint casts for post operative rehabilitation patients.

Occasionally, a lumbar support belt is needed early on in the treatment of low back pain. As soon as you can move more easily without it, the better off you are. Struggling a little bit stops you from becoming completely deconditioned.

A narrow, flexible, trochanteric belt that is placed around the hips will amply support the sacroiliac joints and allow more lumbar motion. Dockworkers, longshoremen, and others in heavy lifting occupations wear these wide black nylon belts around the outside of their trousers at hip level. When they want to lift something heavy, they simply tighten the belt and thus strengthen the supporting ligaments and force close the sacroiliac joints. Recent research has shown that our core muscles also act to force close the sacroiliac ligaments before we lift even light weights.

If you wear a belt tight, for too long you will discourage the active participation of your core muscles.

The following pages of pictures and descriptions of very important exercises and stretches are arranged in degrees of increasing difficulty. If your back is presently still, slightly painful, do the first group only. As your back improves do the second group of exercises.

If your back is pain-free at the moment and you are assured the lower back and pelvic biomechanics are normal or close to normal, then use Groups One and Two as warm-ups for the third group of exercises. At this stage, you should purchase an exercise ball and a book on ball exercises for strengthening the core. Dr. Mark King has published a video tape with the core strengthening ball exercises that are excellent for a home program.

The rule is very simple: Any exercise that causes a lingering pain must be discontinued temporarily. An exercise that only hurts for an instant with no pain afterwards must be continued until it becomes pain-free over time.

These exercises are best performed after a warm-up walk of at least 10 minutes. Follow the instructions under each photograph and do these routines daily.

The body responds to an imposed demand by making a specific adaptation. Each of these exercises and stretches are demanding specific changes to help you remove the shackles of back pain. Just as you cannot learn to play the piano in a few weeks, you can not achieve new ranges of motion, muscle coordination, balance and strength in your lower back in a few weeks. A common mistake made by many is to progress too quickly. The belly of the muscle can strengthen faster than the tendons and the ligaments. When you progress to a harder level, stay there a few weeks so that the muscle attachments can catch up. We don't want new sprains and strains.

Start out gently and build up over months to a vigorous routine. The worse your condition the longer it will take. As the saying goes, "if you don't get a little better at first, you can't get a lot better later". Slowly getting better by being proactive, is much better than doing nothing and slowly getting worse.

Group One: Increasing the Ranges of Back Motion During Recovery

You can only increase your ranges of motion as your pain subsides. The exercises illustrated in Figures 29 through 39 increases the active ranges. Be sure to read the instructions with each photograph before you attempt these exercises.

Group Two: Increasing Back Strength and Supportive Abdominal and Pelvic Structures

Figures 40, 41 and 42 show the first of the second group of exercises that you should start as soon as your back begins to feel better. If you have a good back, these are done as warm-up stretches to more strenuous exercise or a sports activity. Golfers and tennis players must do these to prevent lower back rotational injuries.

The back strengthening exercises are also described in detail in figures 42 to 56. Again read the instructions carefully, and follow them exactly for best results.

The best home exercise program is with a large, inflatable ball. With this ball and the correct level of exercises that progressively get more difficult as your CORE muscles strengthen, you can prevent episodes of back pain from occurring. These can be done in your living room while you watch the TV. Your autonomic nervous system controls the activation of the muscles concerned with maintaining our balance. When you exercise on this ball you automatically use the CORE muscles because the ball provides an unstable base. Many of you will have to start out by just sitting and bouncing on the ball. The last page of this book has a description and special offer for a ball and an online instruction program, which assures proper usage and level of exercises. Unless you belong to a gym where you can use an exercise ball; you really need this low tech apparatus and online instruction for the best and quickest home results. Some doctors and therapists provide a ball and a videotape of instructions for home use. Gym, online, video, "just do it", one way or another. It will make a big difference in your life.

Group Three: Increasing Ranges of Motion When Fully Recovered

Stretching is the ultimate home care procedure for real long term benefit. The muscles and ligaments need not only become stronger, they must become more elastic. No matter how many years have passed since you could bend and twist easily, you can and must do it again. A repeated demand for elongation exerted upon each muscle group for a hold of at least 30 seconds, done every day will show you amazing results. The make-up of the connective tissue actually changes its' properties to a more elastic material. Also, inside the muscles, the set distance of the muscles at rest is elongated; all part of the S.A.I.D. Principle of a specific adaptation to an imposed demand.

Always stretch the most, on an out-breath. The act of exhaling, causes a neurological, reflex relaxation that allows for more stretching to occur. Stay at the most relaxed distance for 30 seconds. Thus, stretching the backs of your legs, may take a few minutes for you to exhale and let go, until the hamstring muscles have stretched their maximum, for that day.

We are therefore talking about twenty minutes a day to stretch before you attempt the exercises. When you are supple, two sessions a week will keep the muscles elongated. This prevents tightened muscles from restricting the pelvis from tilting forward and backward properly. When the pelvis doesn't move enough on the hip joints your back moves too much while it is hanging on your ligaments and a sprain occurs. That's when the stabbing, shooting horrible pain almost paralyses you for a few seconds. With lengthy thigh and hamstring muscles, and bent knees when you lift you can avoid this "dreaded lurgy" as people call it in England.

Figures 25 to 27 inclusive, from earlier in the book are additional strenuous exercises that should be included when your strength has increased and you are pain-free.

Improving Posture

It is worth striving for good posture. The best standing posture is that point where you can raise up onto your toes without first having to rock forward. (Remember the example of this in Figure 13 from the Self-Diagnosis chapter?" Starting from your ear lobe, someone looking from the side should be able to drop an imaginary straight line bisecting your shoulder, and passing just in front of your ankle bone. While sitting, do not slump backwards with your neck forward into a C shape. Sit on your thighs, not your tail bone and maintain a hollow in your lower back. You should be able to place you hand between your low back and the chair back.

It's easy to fall into bad habits, but it is worth the effort practicing the correct ones until they become second nature. Now that so many of us spend time sitting in front of our computers, sitting posture is a major concern. Studies have shown that three minutes of relaxed, slumped posture decreased the deep spine stabilizing muscle activity to zero. Then it was shown that it takes three times as long to get back to normal muscle activity. First of all, get into the habit of standing up every half hour for a few minutes. This prevents a constant stress on the low back ligaments, from causing a detrimental creep affect and relieves the increased pressure inside of the discs, that slumped sitting creates. While sitting constantly, reverse the slump by actively forcing your lower back forward into a hollow that your fore arm can go into, in front of the chair back.

The best and some say the only way to change posture, is by way of your balance mechanisms. Posture muscles are controlled by involuntary nerves, which are not influenced by voluntary muscle action. The act of balancing occurs far too quickly for conscious correction. If this were not so we would be falling all over the place. We wouldn't be able to ski, roller blade or ride a bicycle.

Posture is also an involuntary action which must be challenged by our balance mechanism action. The old fashioned idea of walking with a book balanced on your head to improve your posture is a good idea. You can't balance a book on your head without a good upright and relaxed posture. Do this in your bare feet which will activate even more of the postural reflexes. This is why Yoga is best performed in your bare feet. The best doctors and therapists are using balance boards and rockers to awaken the autonomic reactions that stimulate the muscles, made dormant by our sedentary life-style.

Sitting in an airplane seat completely reduces the hollow behind your back. It actually allows a reverse of this normal hollow. That is why back pain sufferers need to put a cushion behind their back when flying. The same rule holds true on a plane; stand up frequently. Obviously you need to request an isle seat. The first class seats are a little better in that they allow you to lie almost flat. When lying, the hollow disappears but the weight is not descending into the low back the same as sitting slumped.

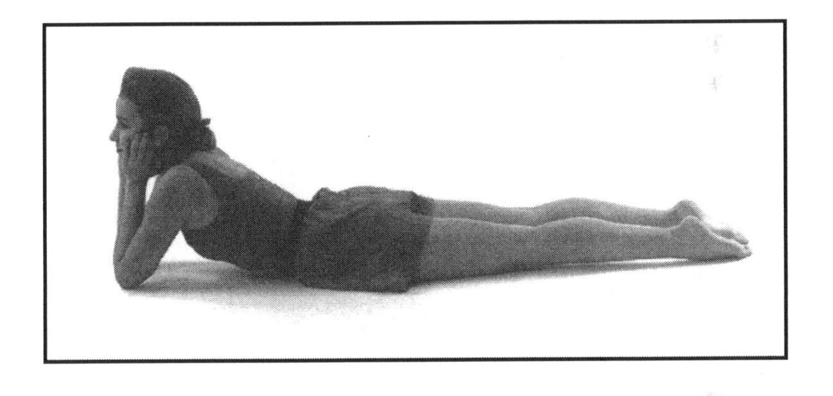

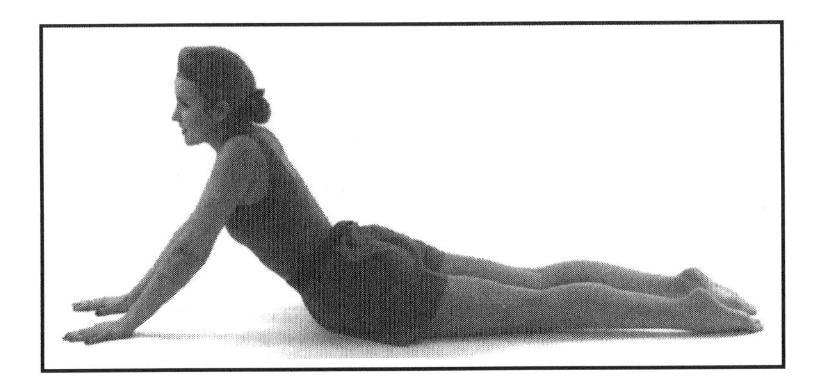

Fig. 29, Fig. 30
You should be able to lie as shown in Figure 29, completely relaxed, for 15 minutes. If you have a disc syndrome, it will be necessary to start with a few minutes each day. Do not do the straight arm version (Figure 30) until you can do 15 minutes of the bent-elbow version without causing any pain. In the beginning, these postures may make it very difficult for you to get up off the floor because of a locked feeling. First lower yourself down to a flat position, roll over onto your side, kneel, and then get up.

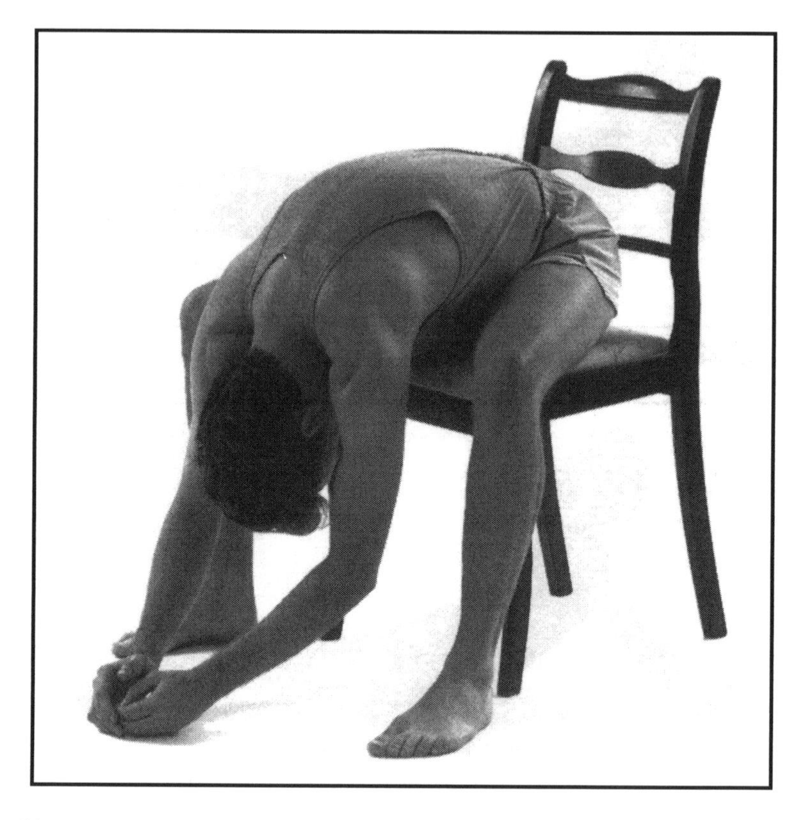

Fig. 31
If you have an active disc syndrome, this position will be difficult for you. Just lean forward to the point of pain and try to relax into the pain very slightly. If it causes you a lingering pain, stop this stretch; if not, increase the forward bend a little each day. With most other back pains, this position will feel good and you can gradually work towards a full relaxed lumbar and hip flexion.

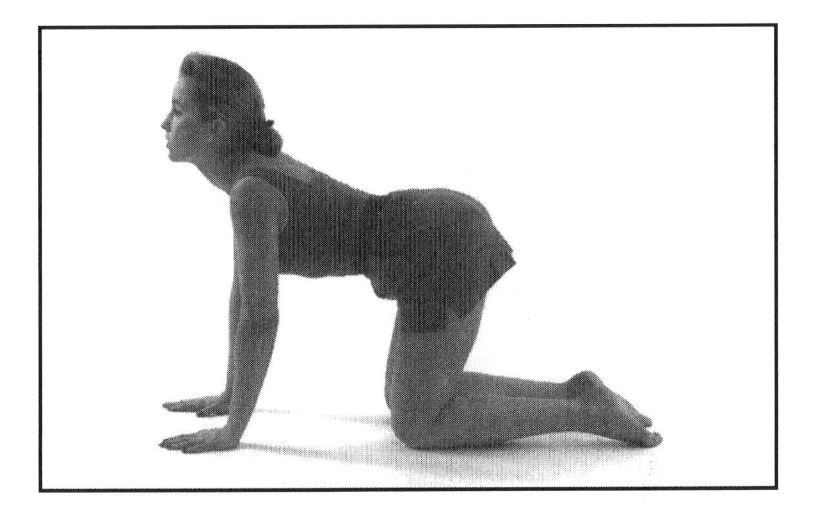

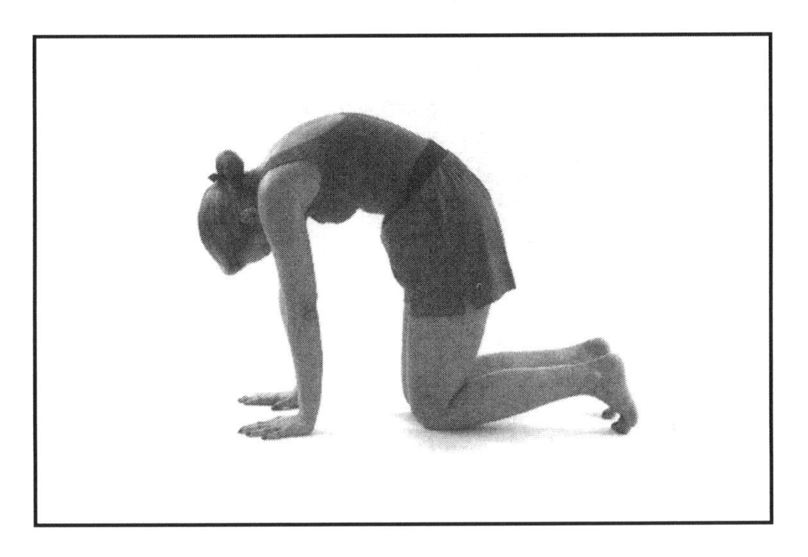

Fig. 32, Fig. 33
First, let your lower back sag, as shown in Figure 32, to increase the hollow of the lumbar spine while you exhale. Inhale and raise your back like a scared cat on the backyard fence, as shown in Figure 33. Exhale and let your back sag as far into the hollow as possible. Hold each posture for a few seconds. If it does not hurt, gently sway your hips from side to side while raising and lowering your back.

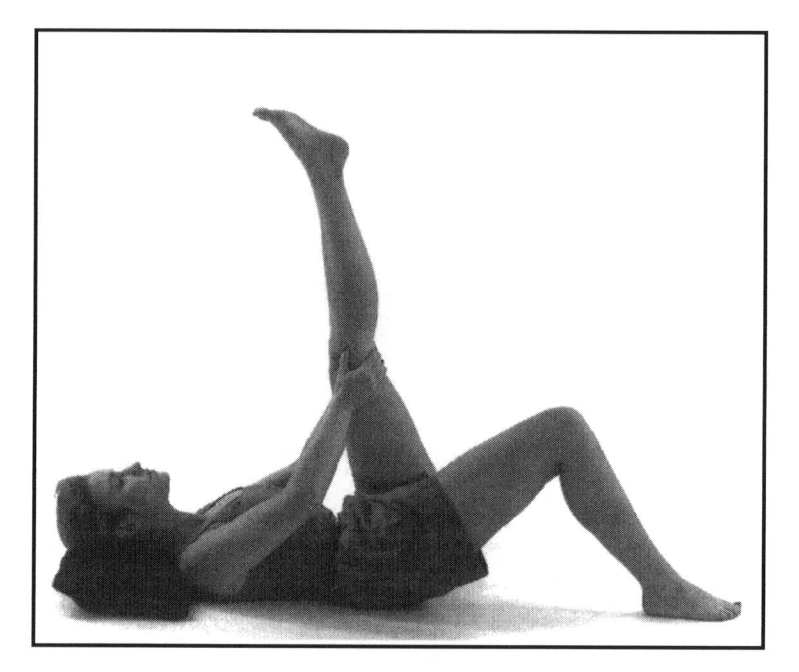

Fig. 34
This is the easiest way to start stretching the hamstring muscles at the back of your thigh. To produce a greater stretch, first contract the hamstrings isometrically, then release. Repeat three times. To take tension off your lower back, keep your relaxed leg bent with that foot flat on the floor. Raise the leg to be stretched, keeping your knee straight. Hold the back of your knee with your hands so you can resist trying to lower your leg to the floor. Hold this effort and resistance for the count of sixteen and then actively raise your straight leg higher, pulling gently with your hands.

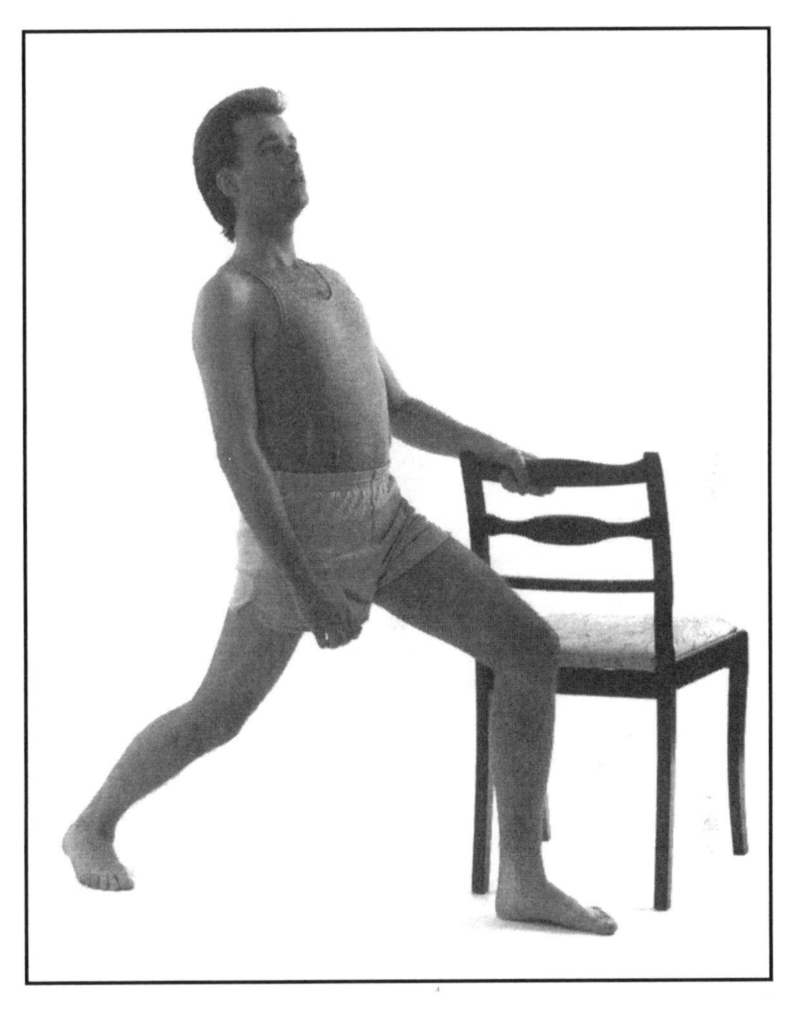

Fig. 35
As with all stretches, hold this one for 30 seconds and exhale for the last five seconds of the stretch. A stretch should not be painful, just a little uncomfortable. As you get better, you can stretch the large hip flexor muscle that attaches to the lower spine even more effectively by turning the back foot inwards and bending the forward knee more than shown.

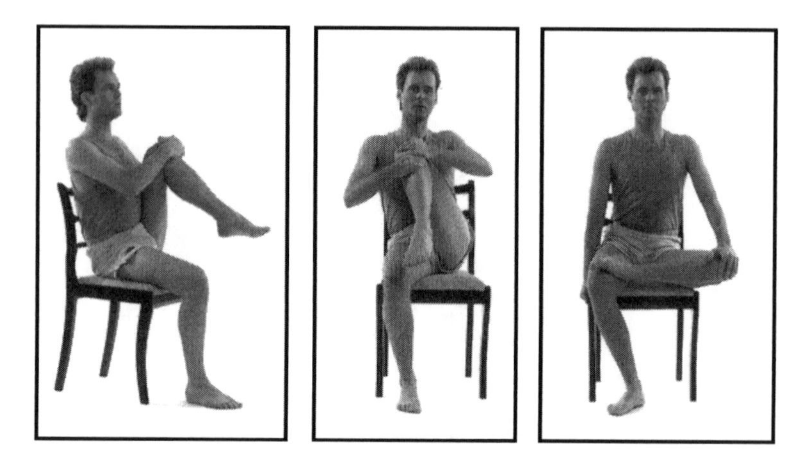

Fig. 36, Fig. 37, Fig 38
These three hip and sacroiliac stretches have helped more back pain sufferers than any other home care I have ever recommended. Hold each stretch for 30 seconds and do both legs. You must keep your back upright for all of these stretches. Figure 36 is a pull straight up to the shoulder on the same side. Notice the hands clasp the knee, not the lower leg. Figure 37 is a pull to the opposite shoulder for 30 seconds. Finally you push down on your knee for 30 seconds, as shown in Figure 38. Remember to do both legs!

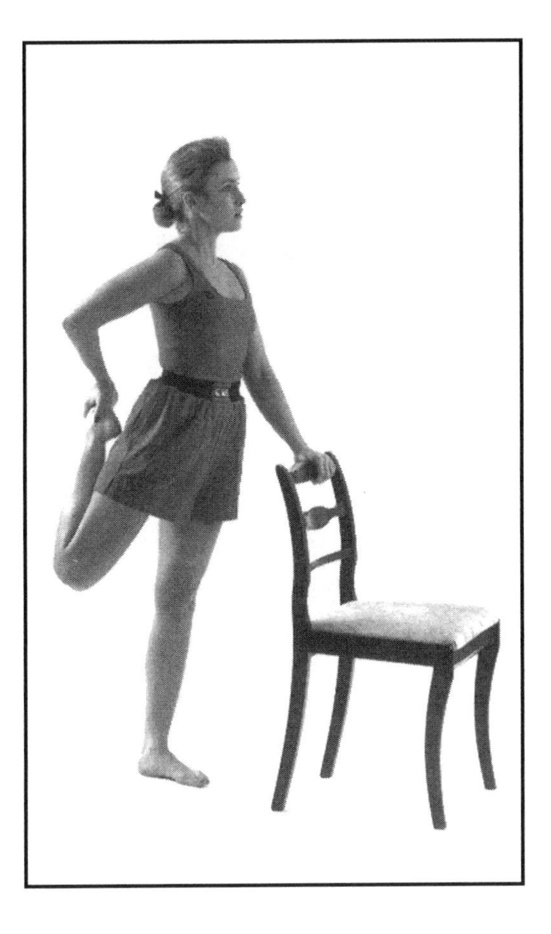

Fig. 39
This simple stretch is very effective for the muscles on the front of the thigh. Stand upright and hold the stretch for 30 seconds. Once you can pull your heel so it easily touches your buttock, add more stretch by moving your knee backward.

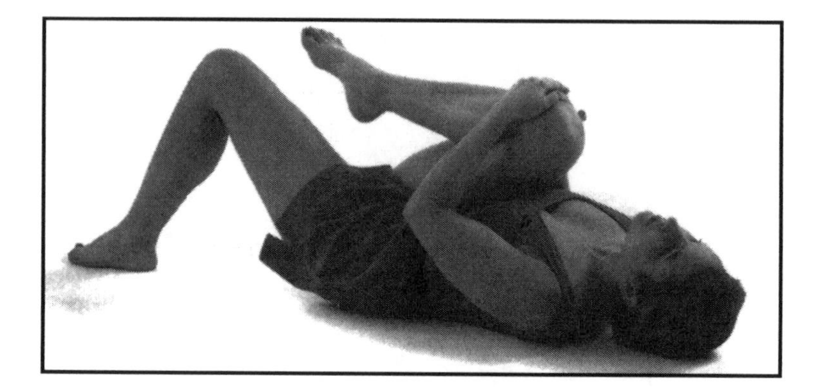

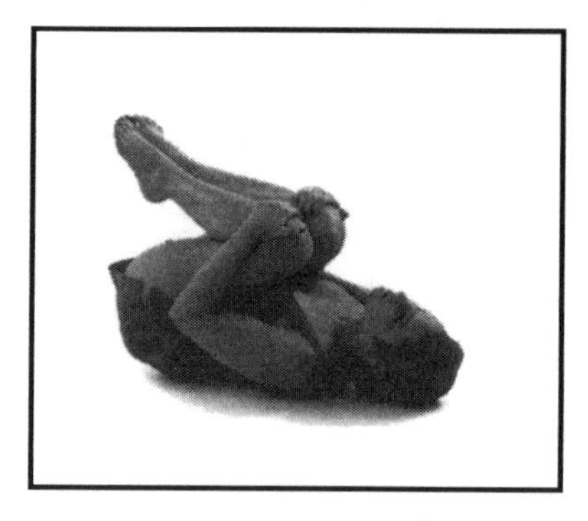

Fig. 40, Fig. 41
Pulling one knee up to your chest should be painless before you progress to pulling both knees up to your chest. Make sure you clasp your knees and not your lower leg. Clasping your lower leg increased the leverage on the knee joint and causes too much forced flexion. If you have no pain while pulling both knees toward you, you can then increase the stretch to your lower back by lifting your head off the floor.

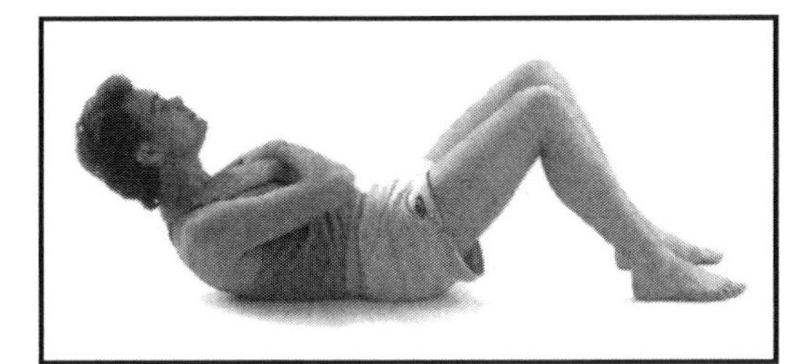

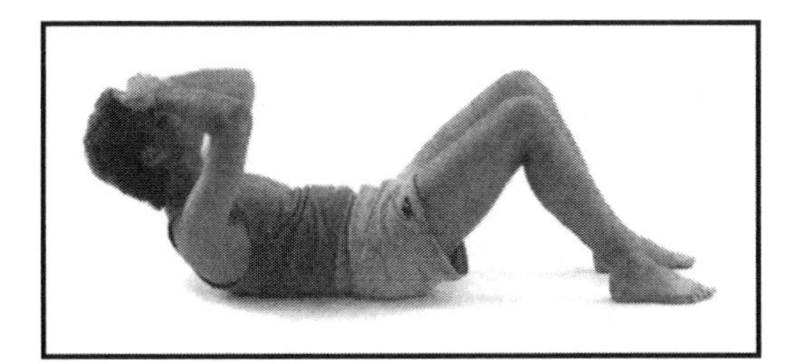

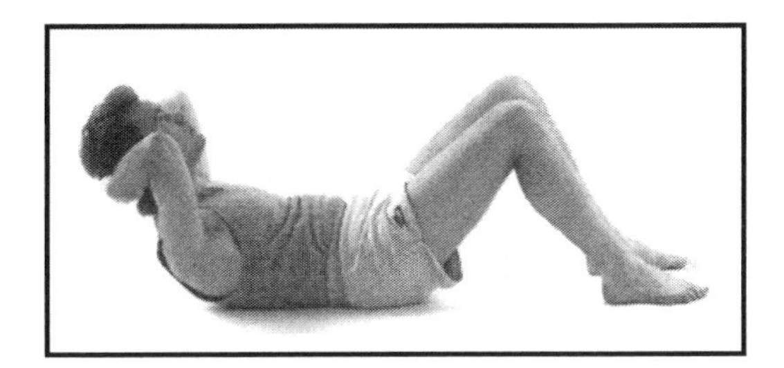

Fig. 42, Fig. 43, Fig. 44
Make sure your back and feet are flat on the floor as shown in Figure 42. Lift your head, neck, and shoulders off the floor for a count of eight and slowly lower back, shoulder and head to the floor to a count of four. When you can easily repeat this exercise 10 times, place your hands on your forehead, as shown in Figure 43, and proceed with the sit-ups as described above. The most strenuous sit-up you can do when your back is recovering is with your hands behind your neck (Figure 44). However, make sure in this position that you do not pull your neck forward with your arms and make sure your chin is going towards the ceiling.

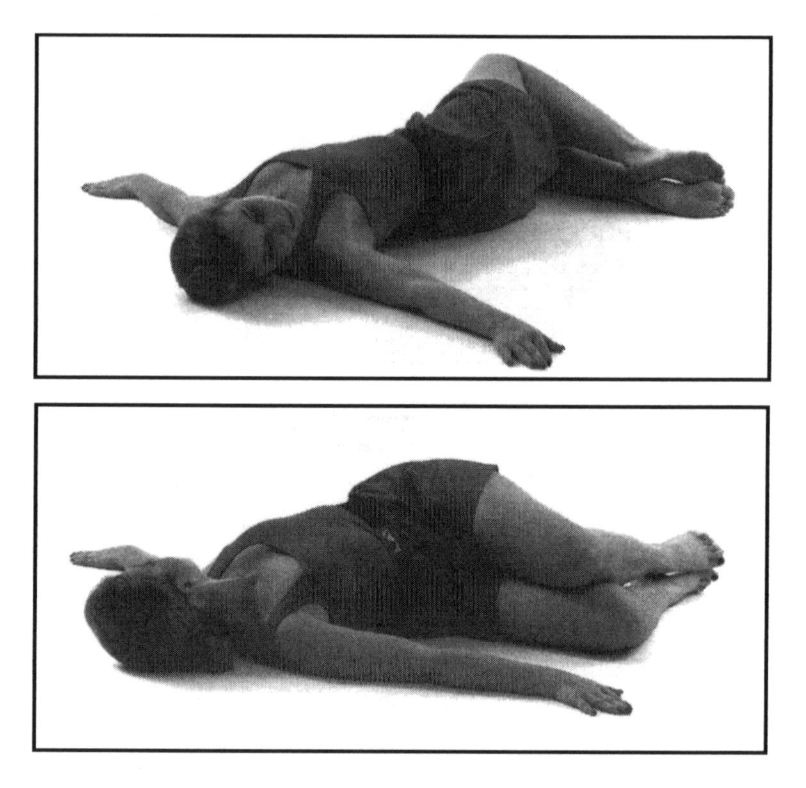

Fig. 45, Fig. 46
This is a relaxing rotational stretch. Exhale as you turn your head to the opposite side of your legs. Slowly reverse sides and breathe out and relax your lower back again. Repeat from side to side 10 times. Do not do this quickly until your back is pain-free.

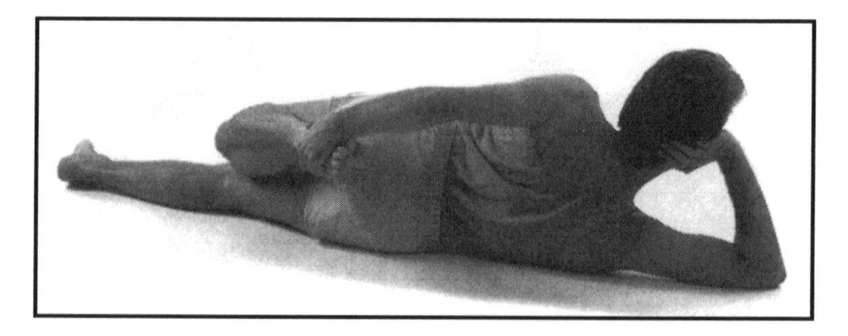

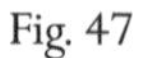
Fig. 47
If holding this stretch for 30 seconds is far too easy, bring your knee back behind the straight leg as far as you can without causing pain on the front of your thigh.

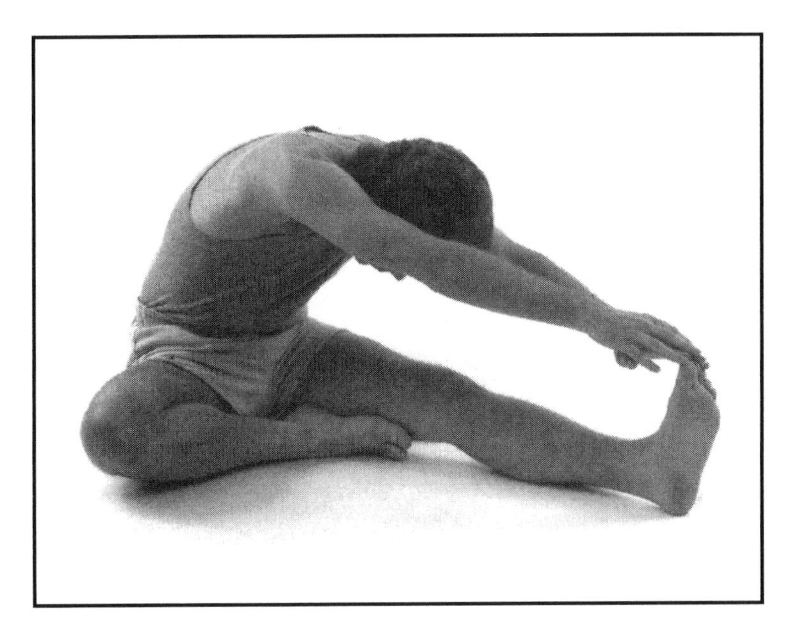

Fig. 48
This hamstring stretch is not harmful when you are recovering because one knee is fully bent. Hold this position for 30 seconds and breathe out for the last five seconds. As you exhale and relax forward, clasp your leg with your hands as far as you can and hold for another 30 seconds. At first, you may only be able to touch just below your knee. Do not bounce up and down! Bouncing will shorten instead of lengthen this muscle.

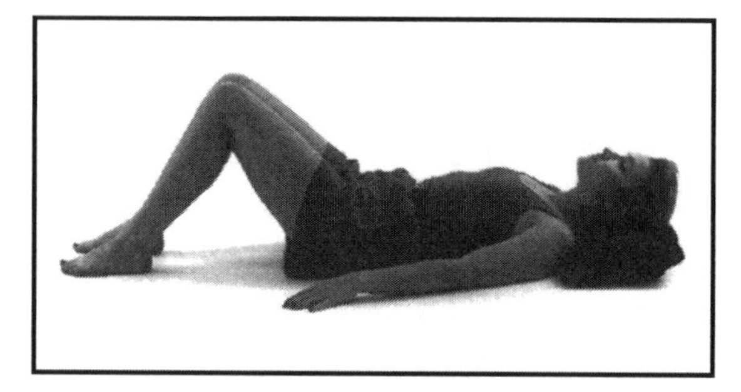

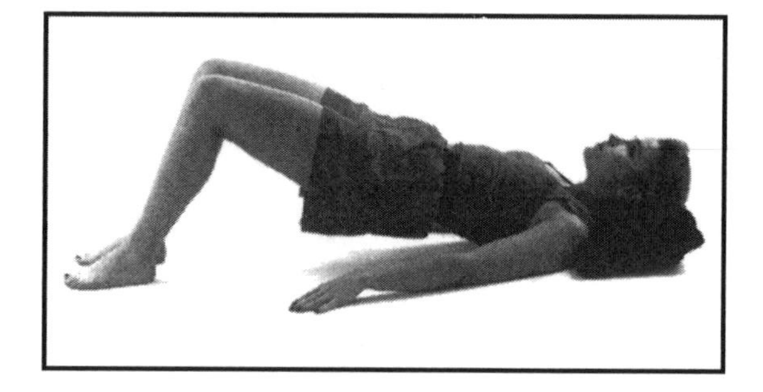

Fig. 49, Fig. 50

Place your feet flat on the floor about a foot apart. Lift your buttocks as high as you can from the floor and hold for a count of eight, then gradually lower back to the floor and hold for a count of four. Build up until you can repeat this 10 times without pain. Between each lift, push your lower back into the floor for a count of five. This will strengthen the two muscle groups that rock your pelvis.

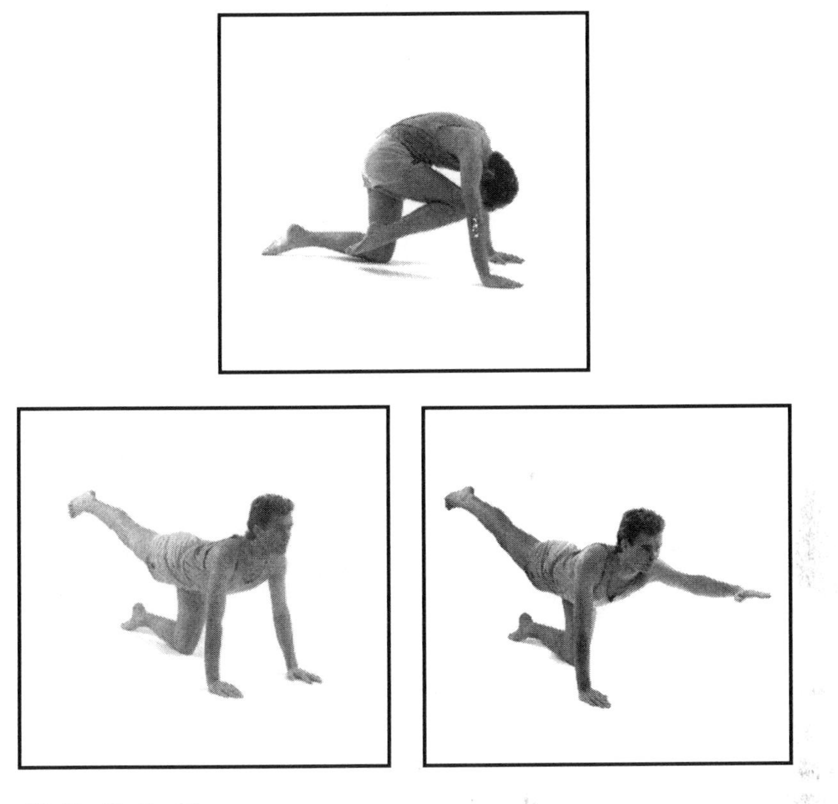

Fig. 51, Fig. 52, Fig. 53
Start this exercise by repeating the action of bringing your knee up to your shoulder and then straightening your leg out behind you. If this action is easy, hold your leg out behind you for the count of eight. Repeat the sequence 10 times for each leg. For further strengthening, raise the opposite arm, as shown in Figure 53.

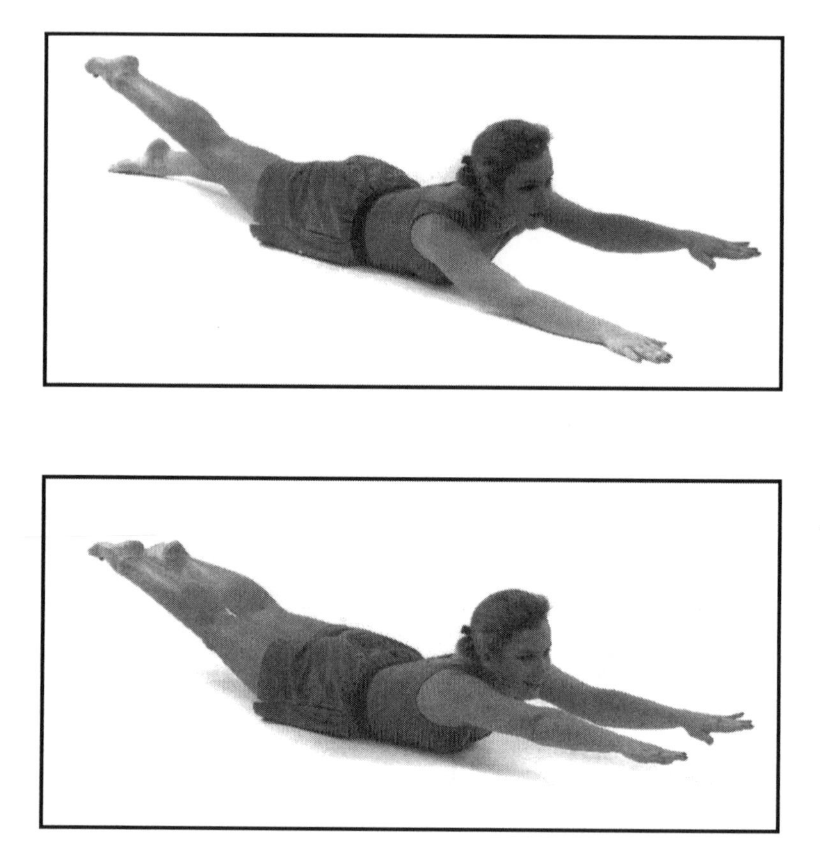

Fig. 54, Fig. 55
Hold the opposite arm and leg up as high as you can for a count of eight and lower slowly. Reverse arms and legs and repeat four times. Raise both arms and legs at the same time and hold for a count of eight. When this becomes easy to perform actively, cross your legs above and below each other in a scissors movement eight times as you hold both arms out in front.

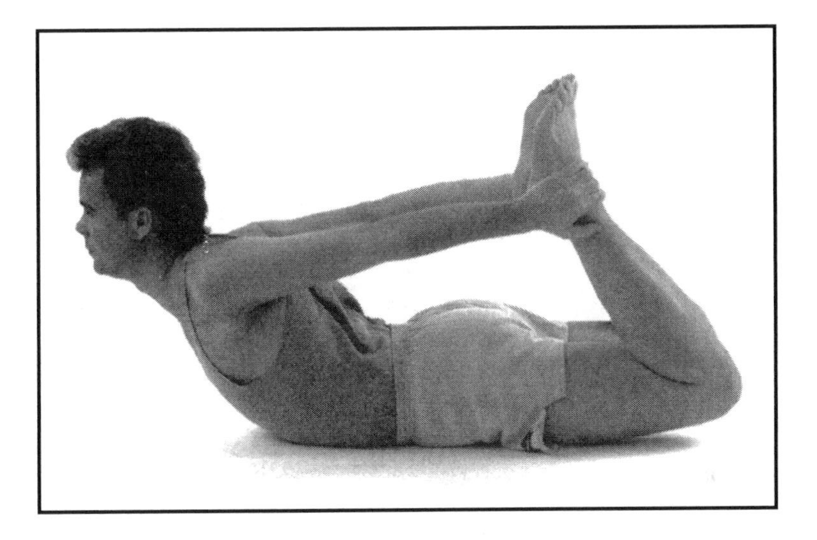

Fig. 56
Once you have raised your head and chest off the ground, separate your knees and raise them off the ground as well. Hold this action for the count of eight. Repeat four times.

Improving Lifting Methods

Always, always lift with your knees bent, even if you are bending over to pick up a pencil or a piece of paper. You can't imagine how many times patients have told me, "I only leaned over to pick up something really light and my back went out".

The correct way to lift is to bend your knees first and then bend forward from the hips and waist. Square up to the object you are going to lift so you are never twisted to one side or the other. If the object is even slightly heavy, exhale as you lift. This is why the weight lifters make a big grunt when they lift. A grunt is a forced exhalation which allows the release of pressure inside the disc.

Heavy lifting is an acquired skill. Never lift heavy objects on an occasional basis, because your muscles and ligaments need to be hardened for lifting. Think before you try to lift something which may be too heavy for you. If you still get the urge to "give it a try", lie down until the urge passes, or better yet, get someone to help you lift it.

If you have an occupation requiring a lot of bending, stooping and an overall strong back, then you need to spend 15 minutes stretching and warming up before you start work. Smart employers will allow this preparation on company time. It will save them more money in the long run over the inflated insurance premiums and increased workers compensation payments, when too many injury claims are filed.

Most sprains and strains occur early in the work day. This is because the cold, tight muscles and ligaments sustain injury more easily than warm ones. Do the exercises and stretches recommended in this book. If you have a job loading and unloading trucks, always warm up before you load or unload, especially if you've been driving for an hour or more.

Reducing the Stress Factors

Reducing stress and learning an effective relaxation method go hand-in-hand. It is well known that people unhappy with their jobs are much more likely to make slow recoveries from back pain than those who are highly motivated to go to work. Thus job satisfaction is most important in reducing stress. A happy family life or blissful single life is the second most important stress factor that one can control. The constant feelings of wishing things were different, having fear, or carrying a grudge can be enough stress to tip you into a pro-inflammatory stress response that you read about earlier. Clear the air in any bad relationships so that your inner thoughts are not hounding or tormenting you.

However, if you can't escape the stressors, then it is imperative for you to learn an effective relaxation and stress-reducing technique. As you shall see, Chapter Six is devoted entirely to a time-proven, well-tested method of relaxation, which I have been prescribing for years.

Many types of meditation shift the body out of the harmful "fight or flight" syndrome and into the calm side of the nervous system. These methods have been proven to work and can be explained by western scientists. They promote a healing response and offer a sense of well being. The act of visualization has also been reported by surgeons to positively influence healing. Studies done at UCLA actually photographed the increased activity of the white cells during visualization as compared to pre-visualization white cells.

Aerobic Exercise and Reducing the Body Fat-to-Muscle Ratio

Being overweight is not healthy, but no one has ever proven that it increases the incidence of back pain. However, it is my experience that losing weight helps clear up back pain. Maybe the exercise needed to shed poundage is the rational reason for the decrease in lower back pain.

Always walk at least three times a week. As your back pain subsides, begin walking for ever increasing periods of time up to a minimum, maintenance time of forty minutes. If your location is not conducive to an outdoor walk, then get access to a motorized treadmill. When walking, swing your arms and take good sized steps. Small steps will not sufficiently extend the hip joints or demand enough pelvic action.

While fast walking does not bring on back pain, you should definitely hold off on jogging until you are free of pain. Being a doctor who walks but does not jog, I never encourage people to jog for aerobic conditioning. The benefits of walking vs. jogging, holds true for all ages. A good rule is to walk at a pace that causes you to perspire at about the 12 minute mark. If you don't perspire you are walking too slowly.

Indoor cycling machines, both upright and recumbent don't usually affect the low back and they are good for improving your aerobic fitness. The indoor, cross-country, skiing machines and the elliptical trainers look like they would be harmful, but they are not.

The most important rule to remember is to stop doing any motion that causes lingering pain. However, pain that clears instantly upon stopping must be worked through.

Stretching

You should make stretching a part of your daily life because there are many benefits you will derive from it, including:

- Reduction of muscle tension.
- Relaxation of the body.
- Improvement in coordination by allowing easier movement.
- Increased ranges of motion by elongating the muscles and ligaments.
- Help in the prevention of muscle sprains and strains.
- Promotion of circulation.
- Improvement in your balance.

Be sure to follow these guidelines for stretching:

- Allow 10 to 20 minutes per day for stretching exercises.
- Don't bounce; hold the stretch for 30 seconds.
- Stretch slowly to prevent muscle straining.
- A good stretch feels uncomfortable not painful.
- Breathe easily, never hold your breath.
- Exhale for the last 5 seconds of the 30 second stretch.
- Increase the stretch as you exhale.

– – –

Chapter Six

Relaxation

"Turn off the stress, remorse, hatred, anger and fear .. Discover the inner peace."

The ability to relax in our stress-laden world is absolutely vital. Some people learn to relax too well. They actually drop out of society completely. However, those with no relaxation skills are almost as unfortunate. Their internalized stress, frustration and negative emotions become a disease-promoting process. What one needs to find, of course, is a happy middle-ground where benefits can be derived from proper relaxation techniques.

Relaxation techniques create boredom in your mind. This is a state of mind, where you're neither consciously, exited, wishful, hopeful nor fearful. The transformation from the conscious mind to the subconscious level happens spontaneously. It is by completely not trying that a meditation occurs. The repeating of a mantra that has no meaning to you is how the mind gets bored or lulled into meditation. While sitting cross-legged, the mantra is repeated under your breath, fully, on a long inhalation and then repeated fully, on a long exhalation. OOOOOOOOMMMMMMMM is a classic mantra. You stretch out the "O" sound and follow with the "M" sound the full length of a long inhalation.

Repeat on a long exhale and don't actually make any sound. Do it under your breath and more in your mind.

To begin with, you will probably fall asleep but eventually you will be in a relaxed twilight, meditation zone that will last 10 or 15 minutes.

If you fall asleep you will still get the benefits of relaxing but you may not wake up so quickly.

"OM" means nothing to us in the West and repeating it over and over again gives your mind no chance to correlate it to anything. As thoughts try to pop into your head, just keep repeating the mantra and don't try to do anything else. The meditative state just happens.

Stress stimulates the "fight or flight" mechanisms which increase muscle tension, heart rate, and restlessness and shuts off digestion, and other bodily functions. (Remember the "Distress Cycle" shown in Diagram 2 in Chapter one?) Learning to relax is a big step in disarming your back pain and the episodes you keep experiencing. The idea of meditating is to shorten down the time your body needs to wind down, especially after a hard day at the office or a personal confrontation.

Autogenic Training

Autogenic training has been around for a long time and was credited to being the fore-runner to hypnosis. It is an auto-hypnosis method of reaching a completely relaxed state, in a short period of time. It requires that you find a quiet place for 15 to 20 minutes a day. It takes a few weeks to master the technique, but once mastered it can be practiced anywhere, anytime, to induce a relaxed state. Once you are cognizant of correct relaxation, stress will not be able to disarm you by piling up and causing pain and dysfunction.

1. First get comfortable in loose, warm clothing. Go to a quiet room. Lie on your back with your arms at your sides. Use a small pillow under your neck and under your knees. Once you're settled, say to yourself: **"I am relaxed** and safe." Believe what you are saying. Repeat "I am relaxed and safe" slowly and rhythmically for five minutes the first day, 10 minutes the second day and 15 minutes the third day.
2. On day four, after the first 5 minutes, add this command: "My right arm weighs a ton." Repeat this in the same rhythmical, monotone, inner voice. Never speak aloud. Repeat this command for the last 10 minutes. What you are trying to do is achieve a true sense of having a heavy arm. If you are left hand dominant, substitute "left" for "right".

Within two weeks, if you follow these steps, you will attain a relaxed and safe feeling in less than five minutes. You will achieve a feeling that your dominant arm could fall separately to the floor if it were not attached to your body. When you reach this stage of progress, add this third command:

3. "My right (or left) arm is warm." Each session should last 15 minutes, with the final command occupying the last 10. The first three commands are repeated in order and in the time interval it takes to actually experience the feeling commanded. This should take no more than five minutes per command after a few months of daily practice.

At this stage you should be experiencing a very relaxed state and simultaneously be stopping the ill effects of your stress. Your back muscles should be unwinding, as should your stress-related attitudes and behavior patterns. At this point, people around you will notice you are less stressed and calmer in everyday situations.

4. When your arm actually begins to feel warm, add this next command: "My circulation is calm and strong." As you repeat this command, visualize your blood calmly, but strongly, flowing through your body. You should experience a warm feeling all over. At this stage you are gaining control of your autonomic nervous system and able to negate the ill effects of the day's stressful situations. One more command and you are in total control:
5. All along, from the very beginning, you have been benefiting from daily, relaxation sessions. Now after a few months when your body does indeed feel warm all over, add this last command: "My forehead is colder." Repeat this command until your forehead feels colder than the rest of your body. You will be calm, relaxed, with your body feeling warm and your forehead cool, all achieved by your own command.

You are in total control.

If possible, try to practice the anti-stress method at approximately the same time each day. You are learning to relax, so don't try too hard. Let go and let it happen. Take enough time at the beginning to feel relaxed, safe and at peace before you do any of the other commands.

It takes months to progress from command one to five. The benefits are felt all along the way. You don't have to wait until you have mastered the whole technique to recognize the benefits. When you do finally achieve these commands, you will not only be more relaxed, you will develop a confidence in knowing you can control your stress reactions and avoid the out-of-control feelings of chronic stress. You can also feel proud of the fact, you have been disciplined enough to set aside 15 to 20 minutes a day, for your own, good health.

Print up a script for your relaxation sessions, like the following. Remember, all these commands are repeated silently, with your calm, inner voice.

1. **I AM RELAXED AND SAFE.**
2. **MY RIGHT/LEFT ARM WEIGHS A TON.**
3. **MY RIGHT/LEFT ARM IS WARM.**
4. **MY CIRCULATION IS CALM AND STRONG.**
5. **MY FOREHEAD IS COLDER THAN THE REST OF MY BODY**

When you can achieve these sensations within a 15 minute period, and shift from one sensation to another, then you can consider yourself a master of Autogenic Training. Now you can use this technique anytime or anyplace, such as before or after a big meeting or settling into an airplane flight, after rushing to get to the airport.

If your daily routine permits, a good follow-up to a relaxation session is the stretching discussed in the previous chapter. If being overweight is also your problem, you may even discover your desire to eat is reduced to more normal levels by this discipline and new lifestyle addition. You won't need those rolls and butter to calm you down while you're waiting for the main course.

A large percentage of back pain sufferers are distressed. The combination of stress management as well as removing the mechanical dysfunctions is essential for long-lasting control of the pain. If you have degeneration of the discs and back joints with outgrowths called lipping and spurring, you can still be relatively pain free. Only a small percentage of disc protrusions need a surgical intervention and these are labeled extruded herniated discs.

Good patients make good doctors. If you have become an informed patient who is managing stress, it is much easier to find the right doctor who can help you become self-reliant. The best doctor-patient relationship for back sufferers can be likened to a coach-athlete relationship. Any doctor who does not help patients help themselves is creating a dependency that is doomed to failure.

Saying goodbye to back pain, means changing your awareness of what is wrong with your back. Once you have the diagnosis, you will hopefully select the correct professional to provide rational, reasonable therapy. Moreover, you will have a professional who can coach you through the necessary lifestyle changes that will allow you to attain your goal.

The first edition of this book stimulated many of its' readers to write and inform me of the success they experienced. Since then, I can be reached at drfaye@chiropracticmentor.com, if you wish to communicate your problems or success, after reading and applying the advice in this book. After reading this book, you should know why you and your doctor failed to stop the episodes of back pain with previous attempts. This second edition reflects the advances made by most of the professionals in the past 20 years.

The bottom line still remains the same; unless you become proactive after your treatments, the problem is going to recur and you won't be saying "Goodbye Back Pain"

READER'S SPECIAL OFFER FOR LASTING RELIEF…

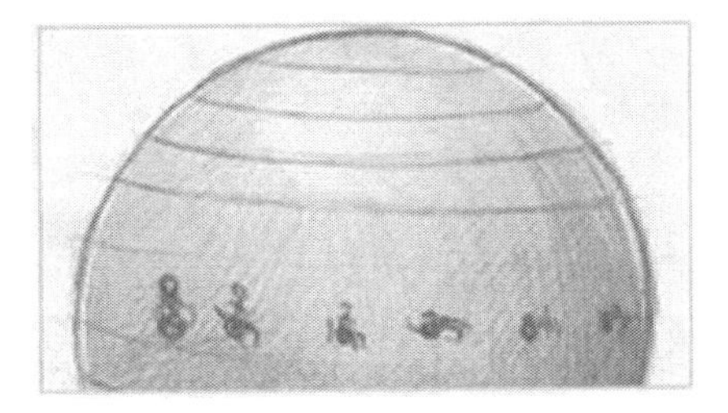

What is Core Ball Training™? CBT™

The first exercise ball with the Elite 18 CBT™ Exercises printed right on the ball. It's an easy reference guide, which will help you maintain proper training technique and an effective exercise tool which builds essential, core strength and overall flexibility.

From the internet, the Daily Online Trainer, video demonstrations are designed to guide you through your daily dosage for a Complete Training Program, which ensures you achieve maximum results at home.

Physicians, chiropractors, physical and massage therapists, trainers, coaches and teachers confidently prescribe CBT™ Exercises to people at all levels of physical fitness. It is so easy to get started and affordable as well for everyone. If you can sit on the ball you are ready to go.

You will start to feel the results after only 2 sessions. You'll become more aware and develop your body's ability to use its core muscles, strengthen your body, and benefit your life.

Core Ball Training™ Benefits

- Upright posture
- Core strength development
- Strengthened abdominal muscles
- Superior rehabilitation
- Balanced rhythm
- Balanced lifting moves
- Stress and pain relief
- Fun and simple weight loss

Gain a remarkable inner strength by maximizing the body's ability to generate power from deep inside the body's centre or "core", automatically-controlled, muscles.

The Core Ball Training™ Program was pioneered over ten years ago by Dr. Joe Pelino while he was working with the Chicago Black Hawks.

Teaming up with professional figure skater and massage therapist Joyce Stockman, BA, RMT and now using their involvement with various athletic disciplines combined with their on-going medical training has provided the expertise required to customize a training program that's targeted to the specific needs of anyone with a weak back.

Readers of Goodbye Back Pain are entitled to receive $5.00 off the unique Core Ball with the 18 exercises depicted right on the ball, and the 1 year on-line personal trainer membership. Simply use the code DR LEN FAYE as the promotional code at checkout. Go to "http://www.coreballsports.com/" and order today!

Refer to the following page for a sample page from the Core Ball Training website.

Printing and graphics reproduced with authors permission: Dr. Joe Pelino, BSc, DC, & Joyce Stockman, BA, RMT, Core Ball Training™ 2008

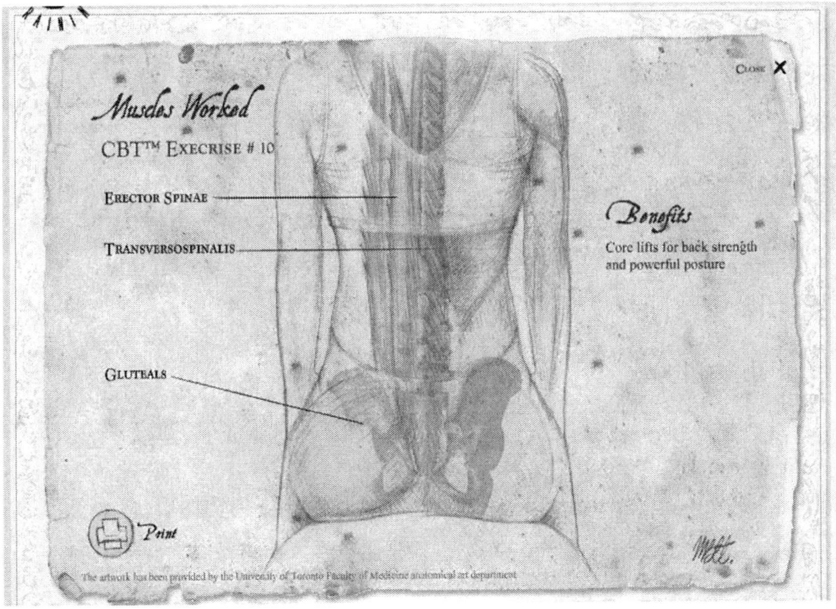

Muscles Worked

CBT™ Execrise # 10

Erector Spinae

Transversospinalis

Gluteals

Benefits

Core lifts for back strength and powerful posture

Close ✕

Print

The artwork has been provided by the University of Toronto Faculty of Medicine anatomical art department

2010978

Made in the USA